Teaching Jumping

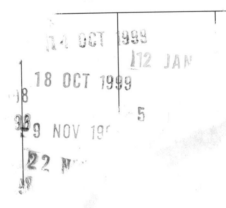

Teaching Jumping

Jane Houghton Brown

b

Blackwell
Science

© 1997 by Jane Houghton Brown and
Sarah Pilliner
Blackwell Science Ltd
Editorial Offices:
Osney Mead, Oxford OX2 0EL
25 John Street, London WC1N 2BL
23 Ainslie Place, Edinburgh EH3 6AJ
350 Main Street, Malden
  MA 02148 5018, USA
54 University Street, Carlton
  Victoria 3053, Australia

Other Editorial Offices:

Blackwell Wissenschafts-Verlag GmbH
  Kurfürstendamm 57
  10707 Berlin, Germany

Zehetnergasse 6
A-1140 Wien
Austria

First published 1997

Set by Best-set Typesetter Ltd., Hong Kong
In 11/13 pt Times
Printed in Great Britain by The University Press,
Cambridge.

The Blackwell Science Logo is a
trade mark of Blackwell Science Ltd,
registered at the United Kingdom
Trade Marks Registry

DISTRIBUTORS

Marston Book Services Ltd
PO Box 269
Abingdon
Oxon OX14 4YN
(*Orders*: Tel: 01235 465500
         Fax: 01235 465555)

USA
Blackwell Science, Inc.
Commerce Place
350 Main Street
Malden, MA 02148 5018
(*Orders*: Tel: 800 759 6102
           617 388 8250
         Fax: 617 388 8255)

Canada
Copp Clark Professional
200 Adelaide St, West, 3rd Floor
Toronto, Ontario M5H 1W7
(*Orders*: Tel: 416 597-1616
           800 815-9417
         Fax: 416 597-1617)

Australia
Blackwell Science Pty Ltd
54 University Street
Carlton, Victoria 3053
(*Orders*: Tel: 3 9347 0300
         Fax: 3 9347 5001)

A catalogue record for this title
is available from the British Library

ISBN 0-632-04127-7

Library of Congress
Cataloging-in-publication Data
is available

Contents

Introduction

Teaching Jumping clearly explains how to teach the classical jumping position along with a simple step-by-step approach to training the horse for all types of jumping. It is essential reading for those taking the British Horse Society teaching examinations, as many of the criteria for success in these examinations are outlined in a practical and succinct manner.

Great Britain has seen a huge expansion in riding, not only at recreational level but also for career riders and professional competitors. However we have lagged behind our European neighbours in teaching jumping from a secure classical basis. We have no difficulty in accepting basic, universal parameters for dressage riding and training, and I believe we should seek to establish the same for jumping. The explanations contained within these chapters should help to rectify the situation.

My inspiration to write this book was triggered by a fascinating two days in Rome in 1995, with Raimondo d'Inzeo. His clear and logical approach to teaching still left room for individual flair and competitive ability, but in order to follow his basic philosophies the rider and trainer required strict discipline. He emphasised the importance of balance for both horse and rider. I hope I have been able to explain this concept and to encourage all jumping riders and trainers to follow a similar basic pattern; whatever speciality they intend to adopt, the basic training should remain the same; a classical balanced seat, in harmony with the horse.

In the 1960s I was a keen jumping rider, achieving a fair degree of success in top level competition. I had some good instruction then, and would like to encourage all today's riders to look for classical coaching which will enable them to make the most of the combined talent of horse and rider.

Throughout the book the psychology of the horse, rider and trainer combination has been taken into account, particularly when outlining possible lesson plans for BHS exams. Study is important for all sportsmen and women, whether amateur or professional, but only 'perfect practice makes perfect'. This is true of both horse and rider and we would do well to keep this at the forefront of our minds and remember 'success is a journey – not a destination'.

Acknowledgements

The author would like to thank Sarah Pilliner for her unstinting patience in putting the text together from my often illegible longhand; Writtle College for providing the venue; Joanna Prestwich for the photographs, and the horses and riders in them for remaining cheerful and enthusiastic throughout. The photographs of lungeing the rider over a fence were provided by Warwickshire College and co-ordinated by Jeremy, who has contributed to this book with great generosity.

PART I
THEORY OF JUMPING

1   The Biomechanics of Jumping

The aim of this chapter is to make teaching the jumping rider easier through an understanding of how the horse jumps. Studying the mechanics of movement, biomechanics, helps in the objective assessment of the way the horse moves. Combined with a sound knowledge of anatomy and conformation, being able to assess the biomechanics of the horse can enable the training programme to be designed to prolong the horse's working life by strengthening the weak areas and avoiding problems.

Centre of gravity (Fig. 1.1)

Unlike the greyhound the horse has a large, bulky body and a relatively rigid spine; the horse is not a natural jumping animal. The centre of gravity is the point over which the horse's weight is balanced. Altering the centre of gravity plays an essential part in effectively propelling the horse at speed. The centre of gravity varies with the individual horse; it depends on conformation and weight. In a stationary horse the position of the centre of gravity can be judged by dropping a line from the highest point of the withers and crossing it by a line from the point of the shoulder to the point of the buttock. This means that it lies nearer to the shoulder than the hips, and this is why a standing horse can lift a hind foot off the ground and not lose its balance. The horse has a heavy head full of teeth at the end of a long lever (the neck) which needs powerful muscles to support it. When the head is lifted the centre of gravity moves backwards, allowing the horse to lift its forehand off the ground; thus movement is preceded by a slight lifting of the head.

Unlike humans the horse does not have a collarbone; no firm, bony union exists between the ribcage and forelimbs, there is only muscle. The horse's body is slung in a cradle of muscle (serratus ventralis) between the two shoulderblades. These muscles allow the horse's trunk to rise and fall or to lean a little to one side, and this enables the horse to keep

3

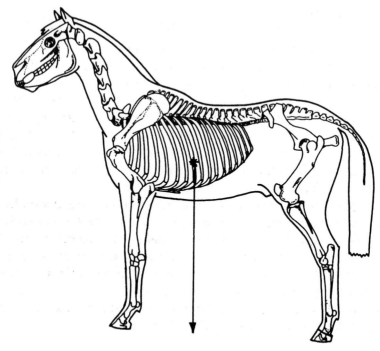

Fig. 1.1 Approximate position of the centre of gravity (*) of a standing horse. (Taken from *Equine Science, Health and Performance* by Pilliner and Davies, Blackwell Science, 1996.)

its balance, particularly when cornering at speed – much like the suspension of a car.

The following points affect the way the horse moves:

- The forelimbs are attached to the trunk only by muscles and ligaments.
- The forelimbs bear most of the weight and the concussion involved with movement.
- The head and neck act as a balancing weight and the neck gives muscle attachment to the muscles which extend the forelimb.
- The spinal column has only slight sideways and up-and-down movement between the neck and tail. Thus the trunk is almost rigid and its role in movement is to transfer the power from the hindquarters forward.
- The hindlimbs have a bony attachment to the spine to transfer the forces of movement directly to the spinal column.

How the horse jumps

An understanding of how horses jump is essential to improving jumping style; by appreciating how the horse moves over an obstacle the rider is able to avoid interfering with the actions that enable the horse to clear a jump. With experience this knowledge can actually be used to assist the horse. Most of the information about the biomechanics of jumping has been gleaned using cinematography; by studying pictures recorded on high speed cameras, research workers in Canada have discovered an enormous amount about techniques of jumping. There are still, however, many characteristics that need to be investigated.

The amount of power that needs to be generated by the hindlimbs when jumping depends on the speed of the approach and whether the position of the feet at take-off allows the hindlimbs to make their full effort. Ideally the horse should arrive at the fence without needing to alter the stride; this is helped by a clever horse, talented rider and an experienced trainer who can lay out jumps and placing poles effectively.

There are five phases of the horse's jump: the approach, take-off, moment of suspension, landing and getaway (Fig. 1.2).

The approach and take-off

During the approach the horse sees, accepts and appraises the jump. During the last three strides the horse lowers and stretches out the head and neck in order to be able to use its forehand to lift and round the back and also to bring the hindlegs well in under its body weight to aid propulsion over the fence. The last canter stride of a horse approaching a fence is quite different from the previous strides, where the hindlimbs are kept well under the

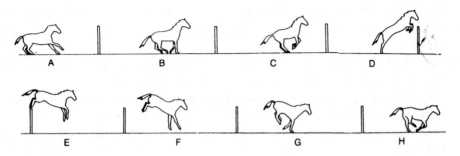

Fig. 1.2 Three phases of the jump. A–D, take-off phase; E–F, airborne phase; G–H, landing phase. (Taken from *The Equine Athlete* by Hodges and Pilliner, Blackwell Science, 1991.)

body; as the horse prepares to take off its head, neck and shoulders are lowered to allow the forelimbs to stretch out further. The higher the jump the more the forelimbs must stretch forward and so the more the body is lowered.

The take-off itself begins when the horse is supported by the leading forelimb which straightens to push the front end into the air. In order to lift the forehand off the ground the horse's centre of gravity must be moved backwards; the experienced jumper does this by raising its head and neck. The forelimbs play a very important role in the take-off, acting as struts, changing forward momentum into upwards push. The shoulder and the elbow are extended by the action of the triceps on the elbow joint, and by the biceps brachii and the supraspinatus muscles on the shoulder joint. A large part of the impetus that pushes the horse upwards comes from extension of the fetlock joint, brought about by the action of the deep and superficial tendons. The musculature along the topline of the back from the neck to the croup also contracts strongly, arching the back as much as possible and helping to raise the horse's forehand.

As the horse's front end is rising from the ground, the hindlimbs are brought forward together under the body to support the horse's weight. There is practically no period of suspension between the lifting of the fore-limbs and the placing of the first hindfoot. The hindlimbs eventually take off close to the hoofprint left by the leading forelimb. The horse straightens its hindlimbs by the extension of the hips, stifles, hocks and fetlocks; the hip is extended by the action of the hamstring group of muscles (the biceps femoris, semitendinosus and semimembranosus muscles) aided by other muscles attaching to 'the point of hip' and the shaft of the femur. The muscles of the quarters also extend the stifle and hock joints; stifle joint extension is backed up by contraction of the muscles of the quadriceps femoris group, while hock joint extension is greatly added to by the gastrocnemius muscle. Fetlock joint straightening occurs mainly through the action of the deep digital flexor muscle.

The moment the forefoot leaves the ground the forelimbs begin to flex, especially at the elbow and knee; these folding movements are helped by contraction of the brachiocephalic muscle which brings the forelimbs up-wards and forwards.

As the horse drives its hindfeet against the ground in order to suddenly straighten its hips, stifles, hocks and fetlocks, the upper part of its limbs (quarters and thighs) travel much faster than the lower limb because the feet remain firmly on the ground until they are lifted by the moving body.

Landing and moving off

The experienced horse flexes its hocks and stifles in order to bring the feet safely over the fence. Some horses kick out, extending these joints behind the body, mainly by action of the gastrocnemius muscle. At the same time as the hocks are flexing, the forelimbs extend in preparation to make contact with the ground. One extended forelimb lands first closely followed by the other, which is placed in front of the first to give a good base of support. The first limb to land is then moved quickly out of the way to allow for the hindfeet to come to earth. The hindlimbs come down one after the other, but before the second has touched down the forelimb has already pushed off.

The strain upon the joints during jumping is tremendous, especially as practically the whole weight of the horse, plus the influence of gravity as it descends from a height, falls on one foot. Frequently the fetlock touches the ground, placing enormous strain on the front of the joint, which may result in a chip fracture (Fig. 1.3). If the horse advances its forelimb a little too far it will land on the heel with the toe turning upwards; this puts great strain on the deep digital flexor tendon and may even cause damage. When the forelimb is placed too far ahead there is no chance of the horse's body using it like a vaulting pole and passing over it. The other forefoot must make a rapid advance to try to save the horse from falling – often the body sinks in front so that the other forelimb is unable to straighten out in time and the horse falls.

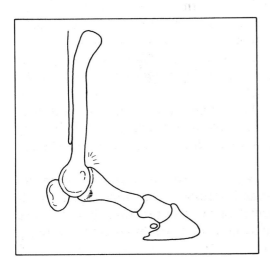

Fig. 1.3 Mechanism of chip fracture of the first phalanx. (Courtesy of *Horsetalk* magazine.)

Horses have a relatively rigid spine and so it seems are not well designed for jumping – the forehand is heavy, with a weighty head suspended at the end of a long neck, all of which tends to bring the horse back to earth quickly once it has reached its maximum height. Horses need long but not heavy limbs to jump well, with a streamlined body. Ideally they should be built lightly in front and have strong quarters, with a well laid back shoulder and sound forelimbs and feet.

Evaluating jumping technique (Figs 1.4–1.10)

Very few top class show jumping horses have a poor jumping technique. In order to cope with the big fences jumping has to be easy for them and they also have to be very careful. Many event horses do not show such good jumping technique; it is more important for them to be brave and fast. As a result many eventers find the show jumping phase particularly difficult. The trainer must be able to evaluate the horse's technique over a fence so that he or she can plan a training programme which incorporates exercises to help the horse jump better.

In the air the horse stretches the head and neck and should describe a good bascule over the fence. In other words, the head is lowered, the wither up and the back round. The forelimbs should be tightly folded as a pair, the horse should not dangle one foot. The horse should be capable of bringing the knee and forearm up higher than the point of the shoulder. The forelegs unfold after the horse has cleared the highest element of the fence. The hindlegs should also be a pair and the horse should be able to open the joints of the hindlimb to flick the hindquarters up and over the fence. It is unusual for a horse that tucks its hindlegs up under him to be able to jump really big fences. It is said to be easier to improve a horse's forelimb technique than it is to change the way a horse uses its back end, a point to be borne in mind when buying a potential jumper.

Another point to look for when evaluating a horse over a fence is the horse's attitude to the job:

- Does it learn from its mistakes?
- Is it bold or cautious?
- Does it find a consistent take-off zone?
- Is the take-off platform secure?
- Are its front legs a pair?
- Does it tuck its forelegs up or do they dangle from the knee?
- Does it lower the head and neck and lift the wither as it jumps?

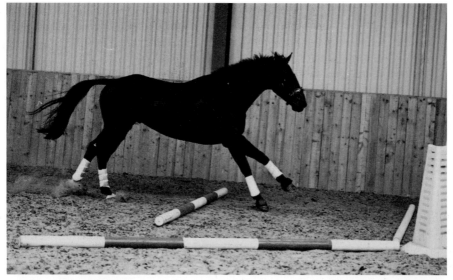

1.4

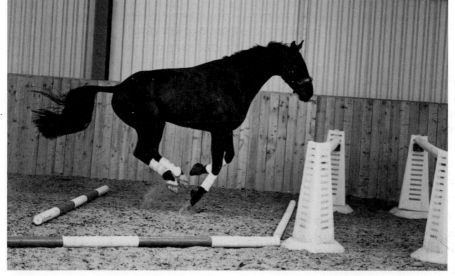

1.5

Figs 1.4–1.10 The phases of the jump.

- Does it give the impression of a 'round' jump?
- Does it thrust off the ground evenly with both hindlegs?
- Do the hindlegs follow through with a relaxed supple back or does the hind end seem 'cramped'?
- Does it land in balance and canter away on the correct lead?

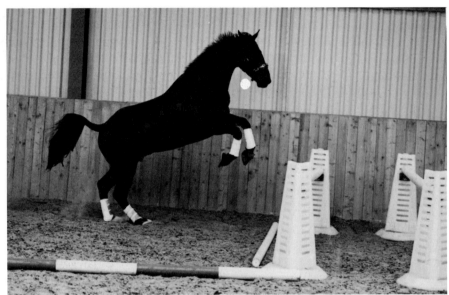

1.6

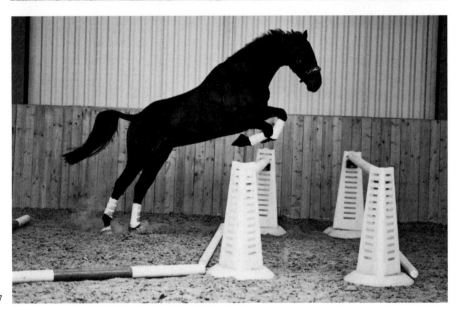

1.7

The phases of the jump (cont.).

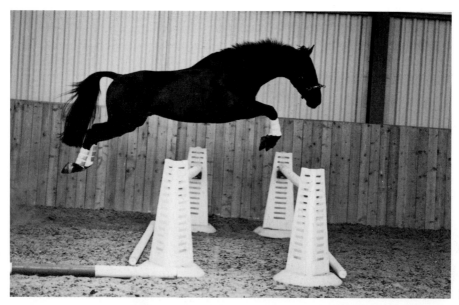

1.8

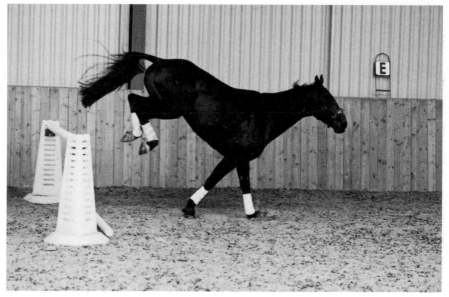

1.9

The phases of the jump (cont.).

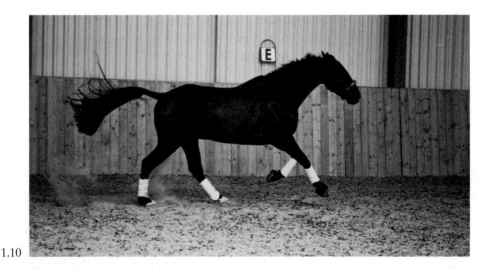

1.10

The phases of the jump (cont.).

How the horse sees the fence

We will never be able to know what it is like to look through a horse's eyes, but we can draw some conclusions from the anatomy and physiology of the eye. The horse appears to have very good vision, having large eyes set high up on the side of its head. The eye also has a light intensifying device which reflects light back onto the retina, allowing the horse to see in dim light. The positioning of the horse's eyes means that it has good all round vision but limited binocular sight (Fig. 1.11). This limits the ability of the horse to judge depth and distance. However, the horse has extensive monocular vision, being able to view a semicircle on either side of the body; thus the horse can see its rider out of the corner of each eye. A further implication of the positioning of the eyes is that the horse cannot see directly in front of its nose or behind its tail.

Horses do not appear to have a spherical eyeball like humans, but one that is slightly flattened from front to back. This is known as a ramped retina and allows both near and far images to be focused at the same time. However, the muscles which help to focus the eye are not well developed so that the horse moves its head up or down in order to see something clearly. For this reason the horse should be allowed to move its head when approaching obstacles so that it can get a sharp picture of the fence before it jumps.

Horses have the added problem of their own nose obscuring the view. By the time the horse is in the take-off zone it can no longer see the fence and is jumping blind. Moving a horse's head from side to side when approaching a fence should improve its ability to see the jump. National Hunt horses suffer less from this as their take-off zone is long and they can see the fence as they take off.

Horses were once thought to be colourblind, but recent work has shown that they are most responsive to yellow, then green, then blue and least of all red. This implies that horses are more likely to 'spook' at yellow fences than red ones.

The time taken for the horse to adapt to sudden changes in light conditions, such as jumping in and out of woods, jumping indoors and jumping under floodlights, seems to be longer than in humans. This should be compensated for by giving the horse's eyes time to adapt. For example, after warming up in a dimly lit area the horse should be walked into the brightly lit school and walked for as long as possible before the bell goes. When jumping from light into dark the approach should be slower than normal to give the horse time to see where it is going.

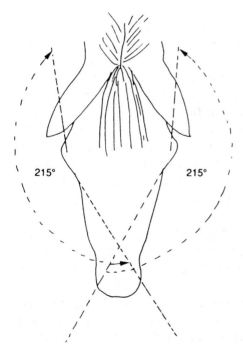

215°   215°

Fig. 1.11 Visual field of the horse. (Taken from *Equine Science, Health and Performance* by Pilliner and Davies, Blackwell Science, 1996.)

Making jumping easier for the horse

Groundlines
This is the lowest line on the take-off side of the fence. A helpful groundline is one that is in advance of the fence. A false groundline is behind the fence. Horses appear to look at the bottom of a fence to judge their jump; thus a clear groundline will make the fence easier for the horse.

Effects of studs
Many farriers strongly disagree with the use of studs on the grounds that:

- they unbalance the foot;
- they prevent natural slip and jar the horse;
- how can 2 cm of stud prevent 500 kg of horse slipping?

However, most riders would disagree, particularly on the hard ground encountered during the summer.
   There seem to be two schools of thought on the use of studs:

- two stud holes towards the heel of each shoe;
- one stud hole on the outside heel of each shoe.

The former overcomes the unbalancing effect of only using one stud but may also restrict the ability of the horse to twist its foot on the ground, for example when turning corners. The latter unbalances the foot and results in varying forces on the outside and the inside of the foot and leg. Generally, pointed studs are used for hard ground and blunt or square studs for soft ground. The size of the stud depends on personal choice as well as the ground conditions. Show jumping riders tend to use much bigger studs than eventers. They are demanding a greater level of control and balance and are also less likely to be trodden on! Event riders tend to use small studs in front when going cross-country in firm conditions to try to avoid jarring the horse too much. The size and shape of the studs used in the hind shoes is dictated by the ground conditions.

2 Psychology of Horse and Rider

The aim of this chapter is to help trainers help their pupils to develop their mental skills in addition to developing their physical ones. It aims to make the trainer aware of the factors that influence the way that people learn and perform, and then looks at how these factors may be controlled by the use of mental skills. This involves the psychological side of coaching.

What makes a successful competition rider?

The cynic may say a suitable background, a good horse and plenty of financial backing make a successful competition rider. However, there is more to it than that. Most sportsmen realise that physical development alone is no guarantee of success in sport. A rider must have the right frame of mind and psychological fine-tuning is as important as physical training. Essential qualities include:

- a strong personal desire to do well – highly competitive people often need strong goals to provide the motivation needed to sustain the amount of effort required;
- total dedication and determination – ultimately it is what lies within a rider's mind that will determine to what degree goals are achieved. The rider of lesser talent who works hard and is determined will often do better than the talented rider who lacks commitment. The strength of commitment may make the difference between success and failure;
- the right mental attitude – temperament is as important in riders as it is in horses; a rider must be positive and confident. Self-doubt and a negative attitude will always have a detrimental effect on performance;
- lack of fear of being hurt;
- physical fitness;
- a genuine feeling for horses.

Factors affecting performance

The factors affecting performance can be described as external or internal.

- internal – those factors that the rider can control;
- external – those over which the rider has little control.

External	*Internal*
parents	personality
peer group	motivation
colleagues	anxiety
opposition	the challenge of the goal
trainers	self-confidence

All of these factors influence the rider by putting him or her under stress or pressure. Part of the trainer's role is to keep the stress within manageable levels. Low levels of stress are often challenging and motivating. However, when the stress grows the rider will start to feel out of control and start to doubt his or her ability to cope and success is unlikely. Trainers must take care not to put too much pressure on riders or they may become over-stressed.

Personality
The trainer must get to know the rider and try to understand what makes him or her tick; this will enable the trainer to know 'when to do what'. All riders are individuals and the role of the trainer is to try to create and maintain an atmosphere which is suitable for that individual. A rider's individual personality affects the trainer in several ways:

- Different people will interpret the same piece of information differently.
- Different people will respond differently to the same situation.
- The same person may respond differently in different situations.

In order to know the rider the trainer has to be able to communicate effectively with the rider, listen to what he or she says (Fig. 2.1) and observe how he or she reacts.

Motivation
Just as different riders react differently, they also have different reasons for riding, for example they may want to:

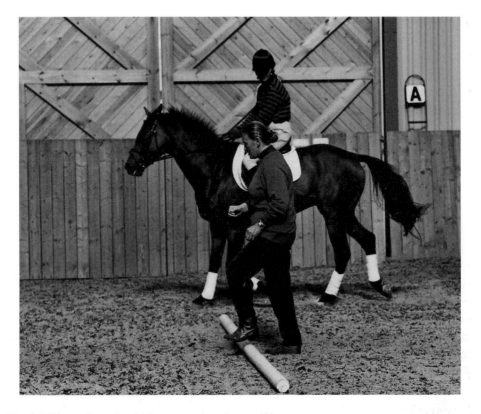

Fig. 2.1 The trainer should listen to what the pupil has to say.

- have fun
- compete and win
- experience excitement
- earn praise from parents/colleagues/friends
- master a new challenge.

The trainer must understand the reasons why the rider is taking part and help the rider set relevant goals; unless the rider finds some satisfaction he or she is unlikely to continue happily.

External pressure from trainers or parents is unlikely to motivate the rider in the long-term, and may actually prove counter-productive; think how many promising young riders never reach their potential. Self-motivation and fulfilment make for a successful performer and the trainer has a role to play in the motivation process. One of the trainer's most effective tools is to give riders honest praise, and criticism needs to be phrased in a positive way which describes what needs to be done rather than pointing out the short-comings.

Mental skills

There are four basic mental skills which trainers can utilise to achieve better performance from both the rider and themselves:

- goal setting
- confidence building
- emotional control
- concentration.

These skills are the foundation for the rider's psychological preparation. Just like physical skills these mental skills need to be practised and some riders will pick up mental skills more quickly than others. There are two ways in which mental skills can help the rider:

- they create a barrier against outside influences;
- they enhance learning.

  It is also important to foster the will to win, a positive mental attitude and to overcome the rider's fears.

Goal setting

Setting specific goals is vital to success; riders need clearly defined goals so that they have targets to aim for, they know exactly what they have to do to achieve these targets and they know when they have achieved them. These goals will be both short-term and long-term. For instance, short-term goals will be daily, weekly and monthly, while long-term goals will be yearly and career goals. Specific short-term goals should be designed step by step to bring the long-term goal closer. In effect they are a plan divided into stages. Good goals have several features:

- They are structured into
    long-term aims
    shorter-term objectives
    immediate goals.
- The rider sees them as stepping stones to success.
- They must be accepted by the rider.
- They must be challenging but realistic.

The goal must be acceptable to the rider. A person will only make an effort to achieve a goal which he or she believes is appropriate, in other words the rider has to accept the goal. This means that the trainer cannot decide a goal for a rider; it has to be a joint decision.

When dealing with horses set-backs are inevitable and the goals will have to be reassessed and reset in order to achieve the final goal. In other words the plan has to be temporarily adjusted. Having this flexible attitude to set-backs will prevent disappointment preventing long-term success. Riders should be encouraged to set big long-term goals and small achievable short-term goals. Many people dare not set big goals because they feel unable to cope with the disappointment if the goal is not realised; this is where the short-term goals are important in building confidence. However, the eventual goal must be realistic.

Confidence building
Confidence can be built up or knocked down by:

- success or failure – success or failure is largely determined by the goals that have been set, and this is why it is important for the trainer and rider to discuss and accept realistic goals. Success breeds success;
- seeing others succeed – a rider may draw inspiration from another performance;
- being told or telling yourself that you can achieve a goal – part of the trainer's role is to persuade riders that they can achieve their goals. It helps if riders can also tell themselves and urge themselves on, thus developing self-belief. One of the most powerful ways for people to persuade themselves that they can do something is to imagine themselves doing it successfully;
- how you feel or felt doing something – the feelings that are associated with an experience are important. For example, it may not be enough to win if that win was accompanied by bad experiences such as lack of recognition.

Emotional control
How many temperamental tennis players might have done better if they had been able to control their emotions? How often do event riders lose a three-day event due to nerves in the show jumping phase? Successful riders must be able to control their emotions so that they do not affect immediate performance. The trainer must be sensitive to less obvious factors that may affect riders, for example they may have domestic or financial worries, and should

try to help them concentrate on their riding. The trainer, by knowing their riders and being observant, will learn when to approach and when to back off.

Many riders find competition stressful and the trainer needs to bear in mind the following:

- Do not change things just before an important competition.
- Do not over-emphasise the importance of the competition.
- Leave riders alone when they want to be quiet.
- Talk to them when they need support.
- Plan the competition well in advance.
- Have contingency plans for any foreseeable problems.

Concentration

Concentration is the ability to focus all attention on one thing regardless of distractions (Fig. 2.2). Riders must focus on what they have to do to win, not the winning itself. Goal setting is important here; for example the show jumper might focus on jumping each individual fence rather than getting a clear round. This also illustrates why it is not a good idea to over-emphasise the importance of competitions or winning.

The factors that have been listed as affecting performance can all distract the rider, ruining concentration. Generally the most serious distractions come from inside the rider; self-doubt or worrying about a mistake. Here the trainer has to be supportive, perhaps pointing out that everybody makes mistakes. However, the successful rider does not dwell on the mistake but concentrates on the next job. Resilience is a quality of all good performers.

The will to win

Preparation, hard work and talent may not be enough to make a successful competitor. The mental attitude is an essential ingredient. The rider must focus on a positive outcome and not dwell on failure. Negative thoughts inhibit effective skilful riding.

The body reacts in such a way as to help a person achieve what is in his or her mind. Thus if a rider constantly pictures the horse refusing at ditches, faulting at verticals or striking off on the wrong lead, then that is what will happen. Subconsciously these are the commands the rider is giving his or her body.

A positive mental attitude

If, however, mental images are of successful clear rounds then this is what the rider will be able to achieve. Taking it a step further, if the rider can imagine that goal is already fact then it will become reality. Top riders sometimes take

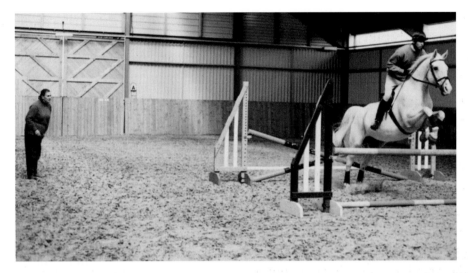

Fig. 2.2 Both trainer and pupil must be able to concentrate.

time out to visualise the perfect round or leading the lap of honour; this helps to eliminate the negative thoughts and prevent doubt and insecurity creeping in. Mental rehearsal allows riders to practise in their imaginations so that when they ride the imagined scenario becomes reality. Some riders will initially find it difficult to allow themselves to have vivid imaginary pictures. However, this visualisation skill can be developed to help riders improve their riding; if they picture success, success is a more likely outcome.

Riders should be encouraged to be positive in the way that they express themselves, for example problems become worse if the rider persistently tells everybody about it. The problem must be identified, a plan to cure it made and the plan carried out. All riders have problems; how they cope with the problem to improve themselves and their horses is the significant thing. Remember, a mistake is evidence that somebody has tried to do something.

Riders must believe in themselves and in their horses, and this positive attitude and confidence is vital for success. Once riders start to let self-doubt creep in, they will lose confidence and concentration and then start to make mistakes. Sometimes it is hard for riders to believe in themselves; their conscious mind might be telling them that:

- their horse is not as good/experienced as the others;
- this is the most difficult test of their career;
- they are an amateur competing against professionals.

This is where the trainer has a vital role to play. Negative thoughts must be banished and the trainer must not show any doubt about the ability of the rider to be successful. Success may be a clear round, being placed or winning, depending on the rider's goal. Believing something can be done and believing that you can do it is the basis of success. Successful riders make things happen by deciding what they want and declaring it in a positive way.

Overcoming fear
It is difficult for the trainer who has never experienced fear to empathise with the nervous or frightened rider; merely telling the rider not to worry is unlikely to help him or her. If riders are to enjoy their horses they must not be overwhelmed by anxiety; horses are sensitive to such emotions and will soon become tense themselves. In order for riders to overcome their fear they first have to recognise it and want to overcome it. They must then act as if they are bold and confident and do the thing they fear in order to destroy the fear. If a rider is frightened of jumping spread fences, he or she worries about it and exacerbates the situation; the more the rider tries to persuade him or herself that there is nothing to fear the more afraid he or she becomes. As a trainer you should motivate action; action overcomes fear. Ask the rider to attack the fence as if he or she were an international jumping star, and to act as if he or she is confident and aggressive. Soon the fear will become manageable.

The role of the trainer

The effective trainer or coach possesses three essential qualities: good communication skills, motivation and leadership.

Communication skills
Trainers and riders have to communicate effectively (Fig. 2.3). The first lesson of effective communication is to realise that every word or gesture is open to misinterpretation and frequently the intended message is not received by the listener. Communication should be:

- consistent – the words spoken must match the tone of voice, body language and facial expression;
- brief, to the point and useful;
- relevant – do not fall into the trap of commenting on everything. The trainer's ideal is a rider who is independent of the trainer;

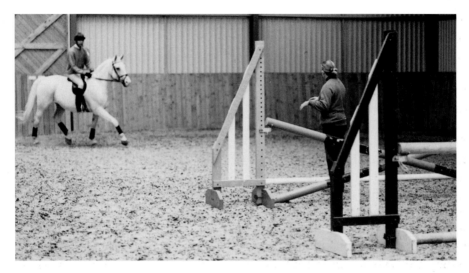

Fig. 2.3 Trainers and riders have to be able to communicate effectively.

- positive – criticism should be about the performance not the person and should be helpful not negative. It helps if the trainer accepts his or her share of responsibility for performances which do not come up to scratch.

The trainer must also be a good listener; failing to concentrate, showing a lack of interest, interrupting or taking over the conversation do not make for good communication.

Motivation
Part of the trainer's role is to motivate the rider to:

- improve commitment and results
- work towards agreed goals
- enjoy the sport, and so
- ensure continued involvement.

How does the trainer do this? Here are a few simple guidelines.

- Get to know your riders and understand them as individuals.
- Introduce new and stimulating training techniques to add variety and boost motivation.

- Emphasise the link between effort and performance; it helps if riders can perceive their route to success being within their control.
- Set goals which will enhance confidence and self-belief.
- Praise fairly and consistently.
- Use role models to emphasise how they had to struggle at times.

Leadership

The trainer acts as a leader by exerting influence over riders. Riders must have respect for their trainers, and this can be fostered by:

- being yourself. Sincerity and sticking to personal beliefs along with your personality are what makes or breaks a trainer;
- being consistent in approach;
- creating a favourable environment for learning;
- recognising the efforts of others;
- being flexible.

How horses learn

When we train horses we modify their behaviour. To do this the trainer has to provide a stimulus; the horse responds and the trainer reinforces the response. If the horse has responded correctly the reinforcement will be positive and the horse is rewarded. Reward will encourage the horse to repeat that response. If the horse has not responded correctly the reinforcement will be negative to discourage the horse from giving that response. In this way the trainer develops a means by which he or she can communicate with the horse.

The trainer must be consistent both in the application of the aids and in how the response is reinforced. If the trainer lets a horse get away with something once but not the next time progress will be slow and the horse confused. This requires that the trainer is thoroughly familiar with the commands for everything he or she expects the horse to do.

Reward

Ideally the training will consist of more reward than punishment. The horse can be rewarded in several ways:

- a pat (Fig. 2.4)
- verbal praise

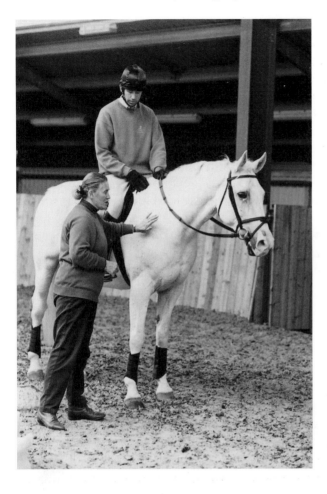

Fig. 2.4 Rewarding the horse and developing rapport.

- a walk on a loose rein
- a treat
- by finishing the session.

Punishment

Punishment is generally too strong a word for negative reinforcement; the trainer merely wants to communicate in black and white to the horse – this is right and this is wrong. This can be achieved by:

- absence of reward – if the horse is frequently praised when it makes a better or correct response then it will soon learn that the absence of praise means that it has not performed well enough;

- repetition – if the exercise has not been performed properly it is repeated until there is improvement. With an inexperienced horse this improvement need only be slight to deserve reward; the trainer should be satisfied with progress made in small steps.
- strong aids such as the whip and legs can be used to punish disobedience. However, before disciplining the horse the trainer must be sure that the horse is not in pain or confused.

Horses must be punished or rewarded immediately otherwise they will not be able to associate the reinforcement with their actions. The aid and the reinforcement must be given quickly if the horse is to learn. Every incorrect step the horse takes before it is punished will serve only to teach it to ignore the aids. However, punishment must always be controlled and objective, never emotional. Horses rarely resent discipline if it is just and they are rewarded when they try.

3 Courses and Course Building

Building a course is part art, part science and part hard work. Course builders generally plan well ahead, are well organised, love the sport and have, or make, time to do the job properly. They vary from little old ladies to burly young men, but they always need patience and a sense of humour. They must be good with their arena party and in accord with their judges.

Courses vary from brilliant creations, skilfully built with the most simple of equipment, to over-complicated, gaudy affairs that fail to flow. Occasionally, as in the Olympic Games in London in 1948 and in Seoul (Korea) in 1988, courses are brilliantly designed and so imaginative that they take the sport forwards in terms of excellence and possibilities. In London, at Wembley, the blind Colonel Sir Mike Ansell conceived a cross-country feel to the course, with water, bulrushes, enormous logs and other features. This set the pattern for the great permanent arenas such as Hickstead, built many years later. In Korea the use of colour, design and imaginative shapes reached a zenith which others still seek to emulate.

Show jumping should be challenging for competitors and fun for all concerned. The most common mistake of novice course builders is trying to be too clever. The best maxim is keep it simple.

Balancing conflicting needs

The requirements of a course builder are many and inevitably there is some need for compromise.

- Show jumping is done for pleasure, or to win prize money or to upgrade the value of a horse or pony. Therefore each competitor wants to jump a clear round.
- Horses enjoy jumping fair, well presented obstacles which are within their scope. This means that every course should be fair, well presented and set at a clearly defined height and difficulty.

- Apart from clear round jumping and horse trials show jumping, there has to be a winner. Thus most horses must fail to jump clear rounds, unless the class has 'time taken' as a feature of the first round. Time is commonly used as a deciding factor in final rounds.
- Commonly there is an audience and it needs to be entertained. The more important this factor is the more it is necessary to pack interest into each hour. This is done by having small classes in the main ring at large shows. Even at smaller shows, prolonged first rounds with most going clear, followed by a prolonged jump-off, tend to be boring.
- There may be a sponsor who needs to be recognised and given good value for money (Fig. 3.1).
- There may be a planned timetable and every effort should be made to stick to this for the sake of the organisers and the competitors.

Limitations

In order to set a course of fences the course builder has to consider the following:

- The materials available.
- The scope and limitations of the arena.
- The labour and time available for building.
- Earlier or later classes, or other events in the ring.
- Time keeping restraints.
- The height and spread limits plus the class description imposed by the rules or the schedule.
- The degree of difficulty appropriate to the horses and riders present. Even with a poor group of competitors the standard of the class may have to be maintained if it is a qualifier for some championships.
- The jump-off, if there is one, will need an appropriate track of at least six fences, outdoors and five fences, indoors.
- The need to fill the ring, so spectators in all areas can see close-ups of the class and also of the jump-off.
- Judges must be able to clearly see every component part of a jump which might fall or be moved.
- Fences must be set so that the horse is not distracted or confused by the arena rails, sun reflecting off glass, movement in the audience, banners, flags, bunting, etc. The fence should always be clear in both its outline and in its nature or shape.

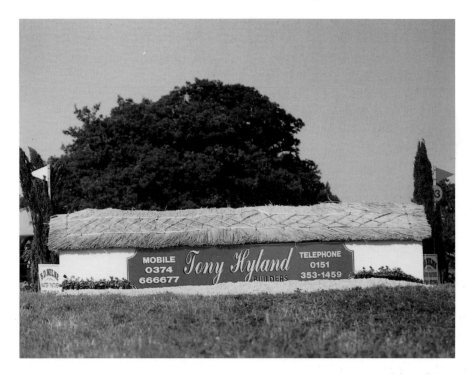

Fig. 3.1 There may be a sponsor who needs to be recognised.

- Every fence and aspect of the course should be designed with safety in mind.

The bare essentials

A course usually consists of eight to twelve numbered obstacles, ideally set in an enclosed space of about 100 × 80 yd (92 × 73 m). One by one the competitors jump this course and the judging is objective, based on whether the horse clears the fences. Each fence usually consists of wings, poles on cups, fillers which are free standing or hung on cups, a number and, possibly, some decoration.

Wings
Wings can be light for ease of movement or large to be imposing. The side facing towards the approaching horse should have the rounded heads of the construction bolts, so a wing is either designed for the left or the right; thus

all wings come in pairs. The feet of the wings should have a concave under-side so the wings stand firmly. The width of the feet should allow the wing to stand up in a breeze but to fall over if the horse crashes through the fence, reducing damage.

Poles

Poles should be 12–15 ft (3.6–4.5 m) long and light enough to show consideration to the arena party, yet heavy enough to sit firmly in the cups and to command the respect of the horse; about 24 lb (11 kg) is suitable. Their colours should be easy to see; grass green is as unsuitable outdoors as tan-brown is indoors. Stile poles, if only 8 ft (2.5 m) long, will be rather light so will need deeper cups to be as knock-resistant as other fences.

Cups

Cups clip onto the wings. Commonly they are made of metal so must be designed with rounded ends to prevent injury to horse or rider. They are usually set on the wing with pins kept on chains. The pins should go in the same direction as the horse so that if the fence is knocked over the pin will not fall out. The pin is also generally safer this way but neither end should be sharp. The cup should never be deeper than half the pole while shallower cups demand more accurate jumping. Gates, planks and hanging fillers go on relatively flat cups.

Fillers

Fillers can be free standing such as a low brush or small wall or they can be hung from the wings as a panel. The latter presents a truly vertical fence and so is slightly more difficult than a free standing filler, which for novice horses can be placed just in front of the vertical line of the rails. Fillers should encourage good jumping and so should claim respect but not intimidate. A black filler may appear like a hole in the ground and cause horses to stop. Strong white triangles, points uppermost, against a dark background may be too commanding for the horse to see the rest of the fence in a balanced way. Strong variations in colour from front to back or vice versa would also be inappropriate.

Number

The number for the fence is generally painted on a rectangular board with a strut to stand it on the ground like an easel. It should be placed close to the wing for safety, and by convention is generally on the right.

Decoration

Decoration can help present a more pleasing picture. Most simple are flat evergreen branches tied securely against the wing to soften the outline. They should not be appreciably taller than the wing in case they catch the wind or take the horse's vision upwards and spoil its concentration on the fence. Decoration can include flowers in broad-based tubs and these may even be included as islands in the ring, off the track of the horse but central to a change of direction. Similarly a few trees in the arena may add interest but must not impede the judges' view.

Start and finish

The start and finish must be clearly shown with flags or two boards creating a line to be crossed. Flags should be passed with red on the right and white on the left. The start is set 20–82 ft (6–25 m) before the first fence. The finish is usually set 50–82 ft (15–25 m) from the last fence, but it may be as close as 20 ft (6 m) indoors.

Designing the track

The track or route is a key feature of a course. It generally has the following credentials:

- The start and the first fence or two generally lead towards the collecting ring, which acts as a 'magnet' to the horse in the ring.
- The first fence is usually a small, natural looking, sloping or ascending spread fence.
- The second fence should also be fairly easy to establish the novice horse on its round.
- There will be a mix of spreads and uprights.
- There may be some combination fences of doubles on one or two non-jumping strides, or trebles on a mix of one or two non-jumping strides.
- There may be some fences on a related distance of three, four or five strides between them.
- The finish should allow the horse to safely and comfortably pull up, and trot a short distance to the exit and walk out. A badly sited finish results in the horses galloping out of the ring or causes delays while waiting for the last competitor to exit.
- In order to keep a class running smoothly the layout of the course may

allow the next horse quietly to enter the ring whilst the previous horse is jumping the final fence.

- The course should flow smoothly allowing riders to balance the horse before and after changing direction; there should be several turns to both the left and right.
- Difficult fences such as demanding combinations or water jumps may be built towards 'home,' i.e. the entrance; this is particularly important in novice classes, most pony classes and team classes. Course builders never try to get competitors eliminated.
- The entrance is likely to be the exit as competitors can find it easily! The collecting ring steward can also act as a safety marshal if there is a loose horse in the ring. The steward closes the gap with a rope and then waits for the horse to head for the entrance/exit and be caught.
- The length of the course plus the siting of the start and finish decide how many horses per hour can be jumped. Indoors, 40 per hour is the norm. Outdoors, a track of 492 yd (450 m) should comfortably allow 30 horses per hour.

Designing the fences

Fences are generally divided into uprights, parallels (both true and ascending), staircase fences and water jumps.

Uprights
Uprights include plain rails, rails over fillers, planks, gates, walls, stiles and so on. A wall generally commands respect but is best avoided coming out of a combination with novices in case they miss their stride and crash into it. A stile 'squeezes' the horse into a jump which may lack bascule resulting in the horse landing a little flat-footed and close to the jump, and so should not be used going into a related distance. A gate is best avoided going into a combination as it may impede the horse if it falls, reducing its chances of jumping the second part clear.

Parallels
A parallel is basically an upright with a single pole behind it. If this pole is the same height as the front top pole the fence is known as a true parallel. Alternatively the back pole may be a hole or two higher creating an ascending parallel, which is easier to jump. There may be a tall brush infilling down the centre of the jump which is then called an oxer. (Once hedges had rails

each side to stop the oxen from pushing through them when grazing.) The back rail must never be lower than the front, or than the brush if it is an oxer. In novice classes the spread does not usually exceed the height.

When building a true parallel, the course builder should remember that the bascule of the horse over the fence will take the horse higher than the front or the back of the fence. Some course builders will build a true parallel a little lower than an upright to make them of equal difficulty.

Staircase fences (Fig. 3.2)

Staircase fences are sometimes called triple bars. They have a front, a middle and a back or rear part. The front is generally low, such as a plank or two with a rail over. The middle infills; it should not have a plank or hanging filler without a pole over it as a pole is rounder and more flexible if a horse misses out a stride going into this big spread and crashes onto it. The back element is a single pole for greatest safety. The rider will aim to get close to the front of such a fence and so the course builder must be wary of building this down a hill in case the horse is too unbalanced to arrange its striding. All triple bars should be built convex not concave. That is to say, the middle should be slightly above a straight line from the top of the front to the back.

A rather different staircase is the 'Whitehead' which is built on an ascending frame wing and has six or so poles ascending over the spread. Another variation is the 'Liverpool' which has no middle; it represents the open ditch on the cross-country and instead of a single back rail there may be four arranged vertically as a 'post and rails with a ditch before'. The flat space between the front and back may be infilled with a water tray. A final variation on the staircase is the 'hog's back' or 'pig ark'. This fence is built like a pyramid and is now rarely used in show jumping. From a competitor's point of view this fence is different to all others when walking the course. The course builder will have measured the distance, not from the back of the fence as is the convention, but from the highest part. Thus the back descending part of this fence is ignored because it does not affect the horse's jump. This fence can be used at home in combination with an upright to build a double which can be jumped both ways.

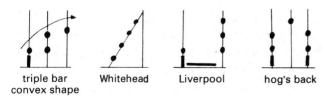

triple bar convex shape   Whitehead   Liverpool   hog's back

Fig. 3.2 Staircase fences.

Water jumps (Fig. 3.3)

Water jumps are easiest if there is a small sloping brush at the front. The back generally has a landing mat out from the water, and a tape or lath to show the extremity; there is then a flag at each end of this line. The front brush in this arrangement is not faultable, which may surprise the arena party as they retrieve the brush and hear 'clear round' announced. This fence may have a single rail, about one-third of the distance over the water, to help the horse gain height and thus achieve the spread. An alternative is to have two rails, one above the other, over the water. Then no tape or lath is required, thus saving having a water jump judge. In this case the brush is faultable and the fence is judged in the normal manner. Course builders need to be familiar with the rules and the difficulties of judging this type of fence.

Groundlines (Fig. 3.4)

When designing a fence, think of it as the horse will see it. Remember, a horse judges its take-off from the base of the fence; this take-off point is generally critical to clearing the fence. To help the horse the groundline can be brought towards the horse a little. Also decorations can be brought slightly forward of the jump, on each side. The groundline must never be beyond the fence, creating a false groundline. With an oxer care must be taken to bring the front rails close to the ground, in case the horse views through them to the brush and is deceived.

Related fences

A fence may be related to a corner or to another fence. Relating to a corner is inevitable indoors, so the course builder should try to get at least 59 ft (18 m) out from the end before the first fence in the line, and 49 ft (15 m) in from the end before the last fence in a line. Often there is not enough room to achieve this, so the fences affected are made smaller to compensate.

Fences related to each other demand a set stride between them. This may be three, four or five strides. The course builder should never build a false

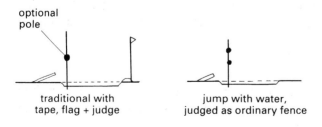

optional
pole

traditional with
tape, flag + judge

jump with water,
judged as ordinary fence

Fig. 3.3 Water jumps.

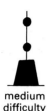 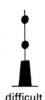

easy   medium   difficult   false   *Fig. 3.4* Groundlines viewed
            difficulty   from the side.

Table 3.1 Distances for a related stride.

Non-jumping strides	Outdoors	Indoors
3	46–48 ft (14–14.65 m)	45–47 ft (13.7–14.35 m)
4	57–60 ft (17.35–18.3 m)	56–59 ft (17–18 m)
5	68–72 ft (20.75–21.95 m)	67–71 ft (20.4–21.65 m)

distance. The competitor who regularly tries to leave out a stride or fiddle in an extra stride will usually have a fence down sooner or later. Experience proves that every horse from a 14.2 hh (148 cm) pony to an 18 hh (188 cm) horse can learn, or be taught, to adopt a common stride pattern. The distances used by most course builders for horses and for Pony Club competitions are shown in Table 3.1. At home, improving their horses' athleticism, competitors may jump much shorter distances, but it is wise for them to also practise and recognise these distances. The course builder will measure from the back of one fence to the front of the next. In setting the distance, the shorter length is used in deep going, uphill, off a corner and away from the entrance (when near it). The longer lengths are used downhill and towards the exit (if near it).

Greater difficulty is created by having jumps demanding that the horse adopts different shapes. For example, an upright requires a relatively short stride to produce an accurate take-off zone and a rounded bascule, while a staircase produces a rather flat bascule. If a triple bar is followed by a gate then the challenge to the rider is to jump the triple bar keeping the horse rounded and balanced so it can more easily cope with the gate. Such challenges, used judiciously, are the essence of achieving the best competitor as the winner.

Combinations
The bounce is never used in ordinary show jumping so the course builder uses one or two non-jumping strides between fences. A combination has

only one number as a fence, but the course plan (Fig. 3.5) will show it as parts A and B or A, B and C. The audience will better appreciate this if it is built to a common colour and theme.

For horses the distance between fences for one non-jumping stride is generally set at a basic 23–25 ft (7–7.6 m). This assumes an ascending oxer going out; if the going-out fence is a parallel allow a little more room, so make 23 ft 6 in (7.5 m) a minimum. If the going-out fence is an upright allow slightly more room still, say an extra 1 ft (0.33 m) on the basic distance. The basic distance also assumes an upright coming in; if it is a parallel it will land the horse in a little steeper, so do not use the longest suggested distance. If the coming-in fence is an ascending oxer no change is necessary. For Novice competitions with smaller fences (3 ft 5 in–3 ft 9 in, 1.05–1.15 m), shorter distances should be used. For fences above 3 ft 9 in (1.15 m) the distances may be lengthened. For indoor competitions deduct up to 6 in (15 cm) for one stride and 12 in (30 cm) for two strides from the distances given in Table 3.2.

For ponies the basic distance is 22–23 ft 6 in (6.7–7.15 m). For smaller ponies (13.2 hh, 138 cm) reduce this still further by 1 ft 6 in (0.45 m) for a one stride distance and by 2 ft (0.6 m) for a two stride distance. For very small ponies (12.2 hh, 128 cm) reduce the basic pony length by 3 ft (0.9 m) for one

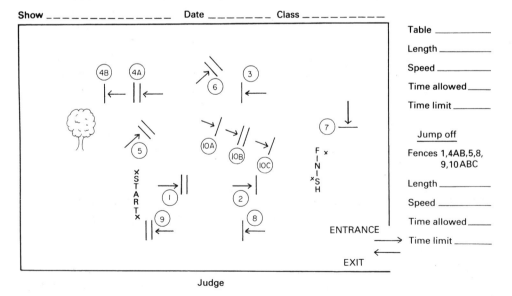

Fig. 3.5 Typical course plan.

Table 3.2 Distances for a one and two stride double for horses.

		Upright	True parallel	Ascending oxer
Upright	(1 stride)	24–26 ft (7.3–7.9 m)	23 ft 6 in–25 ft (7.1–7.6 m)	23–25 ft (7–7.6 m)
	(2 strides)	34 ft 6 in–36 ft (10.5–11 m)	34 ft 6 in–35 ft 6 in (10.5–10.8 m)	34–35 ft 6 in (10.3–10.8 m)
True parallel	(1 stride)	24 ft 6 in–25 ft 6 in (7.4–7.7 m)	23–24 ft (7–7.3 m)	22 ft 6 in–24 ft (6.8–7.3 m)
	(2 strides)	34 ft 6 in–35 ft 6 in (10.5–10.8 m)	34–35 ft (10.3–10.6 m)	33–35 ft (10–10.6 m)
Ascending oxer	(1 stride)	24 ft 6 in–26 ft (7.4–7.9 m)	23–24 ft 6 in (7–7.4 m)	22 ft 6 in–24 ft 6 in (6.8–7.4 m)
	(2 strides)	34 ft 6 in–36 ft (10.5–11 m)	34–35 ft 6 in (10.3–10.8 m)	33 ft 6 in–35 ft 6 in (10.2–10.8 m)

Table 3.3 Distances for a one and two stride double for ponies.

		Upright	True parallel	Ascending oxer
Upright	(1 stride)	22–24 ft 6 in (6.7–7.4 m)	22–23 ft 6 in (6.7–7.1 m)	22–23 ft 6 in (6.7–7.1 m)
	(2 strides)	32–34 ft 6 in (9.7–10.5 m)	31 ft 6 in–33 ft 6 in (9.6–10.2 m)	31 ft 6 in–33 ft 6 in (9.6–10.2 m)
True parallel	(1 stride)	22–24 ft 6 in (6.7–7.4 m)	22–23 ft (6.7–7 m)	22–23 ft (6.7–7 m)
	(2 strides)	32–34 ft 6 in (9.7–10.5 m)	31–32 ft 6 in (9.4–9.9 m)	31–32 ft 6 in (9.45–9.9 m)
Ascending oxer	(1 stride)	22–24 ft 6 in (6.7–7.4 m)	22–23 ft (6.7–7 m)	22–23 ft (6.7–7 m)
	(2 strides)	32–34 ft 6 in (9.7–10.5 m)	31–33 ft (9.4–10 m)	31–33 ft (9.45–10 m)

stride and by 4 ft (1.2 m) for a two stride distance (see Table 3.3). Remember to always allow two strides for small ponies if there is a spread going out.

Triple combinations
When selecting the distance in triple combinations it is best to be consistent, with both parts the same length. A combination will jump more easily for novices if it is built towards the exit. A spread fence is less forgiving than an

upright as the coming-out fence, so for novice horses it is kind to allow two strides to a spread, thus giving recovery space if the first fence was jumped badly. Similarly it is only at advanced levels that a triple bar would be used in a combination.

Factors that affect distances

- A horse going downhill will tend to take a longer stride.
- A horse going uphill will tend to take a shorter stride.
- Heavy going will shorten the stride.
- Ideal going may lengthen the stride.
- Towards the entrance/exit may lengthen the stride.
- Away from the entrance/exit may shorten the stride.

Technicalities

- Find out the exact nature of the ring and the expectations of the class before designing the course and the jump-off course, if required. If necessary ask the show organiser to water the ground in advance, not just the day before or it will be slippery.
- Prepare a table of components needed at each fence and check that they are available.
- While the arena party put the feet on the wings, lay out the numbers to mark the fence sites and approximately check the overall distance.
- Build the course. If the ground is very hard put down peat if it will not rain or sand if it might rain on all landing zones.
- Measure the distance of all proposed courses and jump-off courses; where fences will be moved use spray paint on the grass to mark their next site.
- When measuring the course length, take the track of a competitor being reasonably careful. If a measuring wheel is not available an average pace is a yard; reduce the total by 10% to turn it into metres.
- Draw all the course plans and fill in the technical details, consulting the schedule, the rules and a table of speeds to find the time allowed. The time limit is twice the time allowed.
- The practice area should be spacious, say $80\,m^2$. There should be an upright and a spread fence clearly marked with a red flag or wing on the right and a white flag or wing on the left. A low cross pole is also useful.

- Immediately prior to the class check related distances, heights and spreads to ensure no competitor has made overnight 'helpful' adjustments! Get the judge to inspect and pass the course; allow competitors time to walk it.
- Ensure the judge has a course plan, drawn with the judge's box bottom centre of the plan. Ensure that there is a course plan at the collecting ring.
- With the aid of the arena party, ensure the course is the same for every competitor.
- Raise jump-off fences and blank off others.
- Set the next course during the prize giving.
- After the last class say goodbye to the judges. Dismantle and stack all jumps. Remove any sand so the grass can grow again, or spread out any peat.
- Thank the arena party.
- Collect expenses (and honorarium).

4   The Development of Show Jumping

The first mention of how to jump occurs in a French cavalry manual of 1788. In Britain the Enclosures Act of the eighteenth century resulted in grazing land being confined by hedges and fences, rather than being common land. This led to hunting people having to leap obstacles to stay with hounds. Initially jumping in competition was limited to steeple chasing. A match in Ireland between two hunting men in 1752 is the first recorded jump race. About a century later horse leaping entered the agricultural show schedules; the Dublin show of 1856 included classes for 'high' and 'wide' leaps. Some jumping classes required the competitors to leave the show ground and jump fences in the local countryside. Classes for style were common, but the judging was very subjective and often controversial. The normal seat still used long stirrups and an upright posture with the rider leaning back over the fence for extra safety, and maybe a hand held aloft to aid balance.

In 1875 the French cavalry officers at Saumur demonstrated jumping without stirrups, showing that style was being taught in enlightened places. In 1868 Federico Caprilli was born in Italy; although he only lived 37 years he revolutionised show jumping. Caprilli became an army officer, working at the great Italian cavalry schools of Modena, Tor di Quinto and Pinerolo. He found that the horse could jump better if the rider's centre of gravity was directly above that of the horse during the jump, hence the development of the forward seat. His methods were adopted by the Italian cavalry and riders from around the world came to learn the new style. In 1894 Baron Pierre de Coubertin founded the International Olympics Committee and two years later the first modern Olympic Games were held. The next Olympics, in Paris (1900), included equestrian competitions for style, high and long jumps. Twelve years later, in Stockholm, the Olympics included team show jumping with a maximum height of 4 ft 6 in (1.37 m).

After World War I, international show jumping was mostly for military teams. The first post-war Games were held in Antwerp, with the Italians winning individual gold and silver plus team bronze, showing the strength of their cavalry school teaching. The Swedes won team gold and, as the champions, suggested setting up an international body to control horse sports. So the International Equestrian Federation or Fédération Équestre Internationale (FEI) was formed. In 1921 the British Show Jumping Association (BSJA) was created, its role to promote the sport and to stabilise the rules. Another important event for Britain's horse sports was the formation of the Pony Club in 1929. In the Los Angeles Olympics of 1932, the course builder rather 'over-cooked the goose' as no team finished. Then, in 1936 in Berlin, the Germans won to no-one's surprise. During World War ll the sport was generally discontinued.

During the War a fine horseman, Colonel Mike Ansell, was blinded and imprisoned; there he planned the future of British show jumping. After the War he was elected chairman of the BSJA and Britain began sending teams abroad again to compete. Pat Smythe was the first woman to be included in a team although she was not allowed to compete in the Nations Cup contests. In 1948 Britain hosted the Olympics at Wembley Stadium. The final event was the team show jumping. A course weighing 15 tons was man-handled into the arena and built overnight; unfortunately rain resulted in deep going. Nonetheless the British team, including Harry Llewellyn on Foxhunter, won a bronze medal and became national heroes. Later that year national rules for show jumping were changed to do away with the 'laths' or slats of wood which were laid on top of the jumps to ensure 'clean jumping'. Several years on, the penalty points were changed so that a knock-down cost four faults. Previously a knock-down with the front legs had constituted four faults, while a knock-down with the back legs had only cost two faults. This change reduced controversy as well as the pressure on short-sighted judges!

In 1952 at the Helsinki Olympic Games the British team included Llewellyn on Foxhunter and Wilf White on Nizefella, a horse with a big kick-back; they won the gold medal and brought great popularity to the sport, from both spectators and competitors. Fours years later women were allowed in the Olympic teams and Pat Smythe helped Britain to team bronze. At Rome in 1960 David Broome won individual bronze on Sunsalve and four years later Britain's most stylish show jumper, Peter Robeson on Firecrest, won another individual bronze. In Mexico Britain went one better with Marion Coakes winning individual silver on her 14.2 hh (148 cm) pony, Stroller, while David Broome won his second individual bronze on Mister Softee. Britain's winning ways continued in 1972 with Ann Moore on Psalm gaining individual silver. However, in Montreal our best was Debbie Johnsey in fourth place. In 1980 the British team attended the 'alternative' Olympics where the team won silver, as did John Whittaker on Ryan's Son in the individual contest. In Los Angeles John was joined by his brother

Micheal in the team which won the silver medal. Then in Seoul, in 1988, David Broome was fourth individual, but our winning streak at the Olympics had ended.

Throughout this time the nature of show jumping competition evolved so that we now see longer, lighter poles with shallower cups, which call for accurate jumping. Indoors, courses became more complex and wider rings allowed a greater range of fences on diagonal lines across the ring. Arena decoration also became more flamboyant. Modern international courses call for powerful jumpers of the kind so carefully bred by many other European countries. Unfortunately Britain failed to organise its horse breeding until the latter half of the 1990s with the Horse Database. This meant that top competitors often had to buy foreign horses.

The apparent decline in Britain's show jumping fortunes can be attributed to many causes. For a decade the international team was based on four elite riders. The skills in the sport tend to be based on individual flair rather than a training and coaching system. Similarly, in the parallel sport of eventing, much has been said and done to improve the dressage and cross-country phases, yet the records show that the show jumping is all too often the Achilles' heel.

Although the Pony Club and the British Horse Society give Britain a superb equestrian base, there is no system for the training of show jumping riders. It is only as the twenty-first century approaches that it is recognised that trained skill to an agreed system is needed if Britain is to reclaim the position and respect it used to have in show jumping.

5 Tack

During the training of horse and rider the question of correct tack will arise. The rider may want advice in the following areas:

- saddle fit and its effect on horse and rider;
- bits and bridles;
- nosebands;
- martingales and other schooling aids.

Trainers should discuss with their riders the mode of action of the tack, its good and bad points, and which type of horse, rider or problem each piece of equipment would suit.

Saddle fitting

The saddle must fit both horse and rider. A poorly fitting saddle may be uncomfortable to the horse and cause poor performance. A properly fitting saddle:

- conforms to the shape of the horse's back;
- does not damage the horse's back;
- distributes the rider's weight comfortably;
- does not restrict the horse.

In an ideal situation each horse would have its own saddle which has settled down to the horse's own particular shape. Remember that the horse's shape will change as it matures and becomes fitter. The shape of the saddle will also change as the padding flattens.

The most important principles of saddle fitting are:

- The saddle must not touch the spine along its length or across its width. The gullet of the saddle will need to be at least 6.25–7.5 cm throughout its length. Beware of saddles where the channel narrows as the two sides of the panel move inwards.

- The saddle must not interfere with free movement of the shoulder.
- The panel must bear weight evenly on the horse's back and over as large an area as possible, distributing the rider's weight over the whole weight-bearing surface.
- The panel must be free from lumps and be comfortable for the horse.
- The whole length of the saddle should fit closely to the horse's back to avoid it moving horizontally or vertically across the back.

The saddle must also help enhance the rider's performance and should:

- be comfortable
- provide security
- provide control
- position the rider as near to the horse's centre of balance as possible to enable the rider to be in balance with the horse.

Examining a saddle

The tree should be tested for breakage and damage which may be on one or both sides of the tree. If the front arch is damaged it may widen and come down on the withers. To test the tree place the hands either side of the pommel and try to widen and move the arch, or hold the cantle with both hands and grip the pommel between the knees, squeezing the knees together; any movement or clicking sound indicates damage. If the waist is damaged there will be movement when the pommel is placed against the stomach and the cantle pressed up towards the pommel. There is always some give in the seat of a spring tree saddle but it should spring back into place when released. The cantle should be rigid and any movement would indicate damage. The saddle should be examined underneath for uneven padding or outline and then placed on a saddlehorse to check that it sits evenly.

Once on the horse the width of the gullet should be checked; there must not be any pressure close to the vertebrae. The saddle should sit evenly and level with no tilt towards cantle or pommel which will unbalance the rider. The rider's weight should be evenly distributed over the lumbar muscles but not the loins and the saddle must not interfere with movement of the shoulder. Many forward-cut general purpose or jumping saddles sit over the horse's shoulder and once the horse moves the saddle is pushed back; it will then tend to tilt back, placing pressure on the loins.

Once the rider is sitting on the horse it should be possible to place three fingers under the pommel. There must be ample clearance under the cantle and along the gullet and daylight along the gullet viewed from behind. The saddle must not rock from front to back as this indicates that the pressure is not being evenly spread along the length of the saddle. The cross-country saddle should allow enough room for the rider to be able to sit back at drop fences and sit forward up steps and banks. Deep seated saddles with thigh and knee rolls may not allow this movement.

Numnahs and pads

There is a huge variety of numnahs, saddlecloths and pads to go under the saddle. Purists would say that none of these are necessary if the saddle fits the horse properly. Thick numnahs can have the effect of making the saddle too narrow for the horse. However, in the real world such things may be needed. Gel pads are often used under dressage saddles to try to disperse the weight of the rider more evenly rather than to compensate for an ill-fitting saddle. Pads can also be used to raise the back of the saddle if the pommel is prone to tipping back. Non-slip pads can help prevent the saddle slipping back, especially useful in the fit event horse.

Bits and bridles

In theory the ultimately well trained horse should only ever need to be ridden in a snaffle bit. However, this is not an ideal world and, particularly when reschooling horses, the trainer may have to select an alternative bit. Types of bridle include:

- the snaffle
- the double bridle
- the pelham
- the gag
- the bitless bridle.

Under different competition rules some bits or bridling arrangements may not be allowed, particularly in dressage and Pony Club show jumping. It is one of the trainer's responsibilities to know the rules on bitting that may affect his or her individual client.

The action of bits
The bit acts on one or more of seven parts of the horse's head:

- corners of the mouth
- bars of the mouth
- tongue
- poll
- chin groove
- nose
- roof of the mouth.

The action of the bit is affected by:

- the shape of the bit;
- the shape of the horse's mouth;
- how the horse carries its head and how the rider carries his or her hands;
- martingales, nosebands and other devices.

The snaffle (Fig. 5.1)
The snaffle is the most straightforward bit with either a jointed or straight mouthpiece; it acts on the corners of the mouth with an upwards action, thus raising the horse's head. The jointed mouthpiece has a more direct squeezing action while the straight mouthpiece gives more action on the tongue. However, as the horse learns to accept the bit and flexes at the poll the snaffle acts increasingly on the lower jaw; a drop noseband can accentuate this action. There are many types of snaffle varying in action and severity.

- The loose ring snaffle encourages the horse to mouth the bit and salivate, resulting in a softer contact. Generally, a bit with a thick mouthpiece, such as the German snaffle, is mild as it spreads the pressure over a larger area while thin mouthpieces are more severe.
- The eggbutt snaffle has a more direct action but may encourage the horse to lean on the bit; constant pressure will reduce the blood supply to the horse's mouth resulting in a poor contact. However, fussy mouthed horses may go well in a mild, thick eggbutt while a thin eggbutt is useful for strong horses.

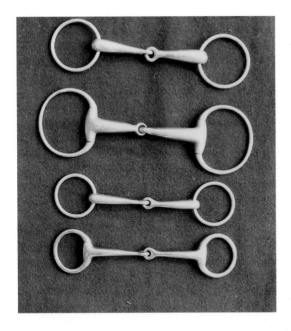

Fig. 5.1 A selection of snaffle bits. From top: jointed German loose ring; jointed German eggbutt; loose ring bridoon; eggbutt bridoon.

- A horse that moves the bit too much may go well in a Fulmer snaffle which has cheeks secured to the cheekpieces by short straps called cheek retainers.
- The French link has a curved spatula in the centre which allows more room for the tongue and reduces the 'nutcracker' action.
- The hanging cheek snaffle or filet baucher is suspended in the horse's mouth, allowing more room for the tongue.
- Rubber and synthetic bits are useful for young horses that may resent a metal mouthpiece and horses that are reluctant to take the bit. Straight-bar and mullen mouth varieties are particularly mild.
- The Doctor Bristol has a flat, angled plate in the centre of the mouthpiece.
- The twisted snaffle has a twisted mouthpiece.
- The Cherry roller and Magenis have rollers on the mouthpiece.
- The Waterford and W-mouth have extra joints on the mouthpiece (Fig. 5.2).

The last four types of snaffle are more severe.

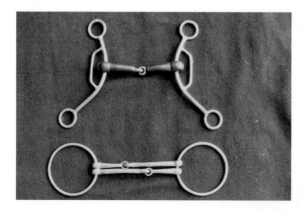

Fig. 5.2 top: American gag; *bottom*: W-mouth snaffle.

The double bridle (Fig. 5.3)

The double bridle consists of a curb bit used in conjunction with a snaffle or bridoon. This sophisticated arrangement works on many areas of the horse's head, giving a fine degree of control. This means that a double bridle should only be used by trained riders on horses of an appropriate level of training.

The bridoon is normally jointed and is thinner and lighter than a snaffle. The curb bit (Fig. 5.4) is unjointed with an upward curve called a port which accommodates the tongue so that the bit can work directly on the bars of the mouth. A long cheeked curb bit is more severe than one with short cheeks as the amount of leverage is much increased. The bridoon acts on the lips and corners of the mouth to place the horse's head while the curb acts on the bars of the mouth, the poll and the chin groove to flex the poll.

The Weymouth curb bit may have fixed cheeks, used in conjunction with an eggbutt bridoon, or a slide mouth, used with a loose ring bridoon. The curb chain should be adjusted so that it comes into play when the bit is at a 45° angle to the mouth. The curb chain may be of metal, elastic or leather, depending on the severity required. Rubber and sheepskin covers for metal curb chains are also available.

The pelham

The pelham is a compromise between the snaffle and the double bridle, being a curb bit with one mouthpiece and a top snaffle rein and a bottom curb rein. The action is on the corners of the mouth (snaffle rein), poll and chin groove (curb rein), but the action tends to be indistinct, particularly

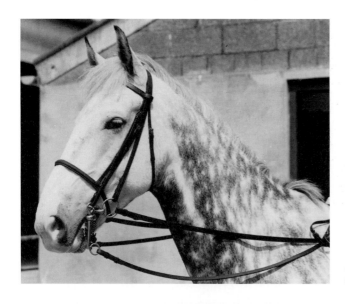

Fig. 5.3 A double bridle correctly fitted.

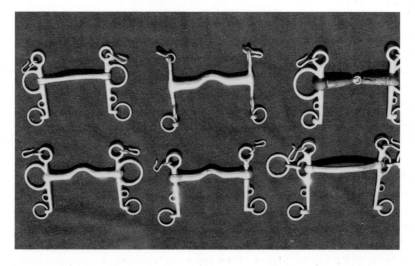

Fig. 5.4 A selection of curb bits. *from top, left to right*: mullen mouth pelham; fixed cheek Weymouth; jointed rubber pelham; Hartwell pelham with port; slide cheek Weymouth; Rugby pelham.

when roundings, which allow a single rein to be used, are employed. The mouthpiece may be straight or jointed and a vulcanite pelham, with its mild mouthpiece and curb action, is often useful for horses with good mouths that are strong, for example cross-country. Attaching the curb chain through the

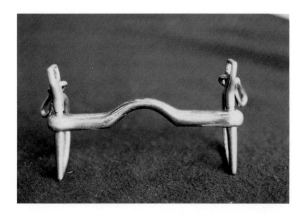

Fig. 5.5 Kimblewick.

top rings of the bit allows the curb to have a more direct action and helps stop the curb chain rising up out of the chin groove.

An important member of the pelham group is the Kimblewick (Fig. 5.5) which uses a single rein and is frequently seen on strong ponies. However, horses can learn to lean on this bit and it should not be overused.

The gag

The gag is a type of snaffle, but the rings of the bit have holes in them allowing an extended cheekpiece to pass through and attach to the rein. This means that when the reins are pulled the bit is pulled up in the horse's mouth encouraging the horse to raise its head. However, with some horses the strong poll pressure may serve to lower the horse's head further. The gag usually has a second rein attached to the bit ring in normal fashion so that the gag rein need only be used when necessary. The gag can be made more severe by having rollers on the mouthpiece.

The American gag (Fig. 5.2) exerts powerful poll pressure which tends to lower the head. With a synthetic straight mouthpiece it is useful for horses that are strong but have good mouths, while the jointed metal version is more severe. The Dutch gag or three ring gag also employs considerable but, in this case, variable poll pressure. In this respect both these bits have slightly misleading names as gags are often associated with raising the head.

The bitless bridle

Bitless bridles act on the horse's nose and chin groove and are useful for horses with mouth problems. However, they can be severe and should be used with care. The nose and curb pieces must be well padded to avoid rubbing.

Nosebands

Drop noseband
The drop noseband fits around the nose below the bit and is designed to prevent the horse opening its mouth and thus evading the bit. It should be fitted so that the front lies on the bony part of the nose; if too low it will interfere with breathing. The nosepiece should be attached to the cheeks to prevent it flopping downwards onto the horse's nostrils. It must not be fitted too tightly and must allow flexion and movement of the jaw. Frequently the front strap is too long, the buckle strap is too long, the front drops down or the headpiece is too long.

Grakle noseband (Fig. 5.6)
The grakle noseband has two straps which cross over the nose and below the bit in a figure-of-eight. It is designed to prevent the horse crossing its jaw. The design makes it less likely to affect breathing. It is fitted so that the headpiece ends just above the facial crest and the two straps are stitched together or passes through a leather pad.

Flash noseband (Fig. 5.7)
The flash noseband consists of a cavesson plus a strap which passes through a loop on the front of the noseband and does up under the bit. Again it is less likely to affect the horse's breathing and it also allows the use of a standing martingale.

Kineton noseband (Fig. 5.8)
The Kineton noseband transfers some of the bit pressure to the nose and is used on strong horses. It consists of two metal loops attached to each other by an adjustable strap. Each loop fits around the bit ring next to the horse's face so that the centre strap rests on the bony part of the nose. When the reins are pulled the pull is transferred via the bit to the nose.

Martingales and other schooling aids

Competition rules frequently limit the use of martingales and schooling aids. These rules often apply at the venue as well as during the competition. Most schooling aids are designed to teach the horse to lower and stretch its head and neck, thus stretching the muscles of the back and allowing the horse to engage the hindquarters. Schooling aids are used throughout much of

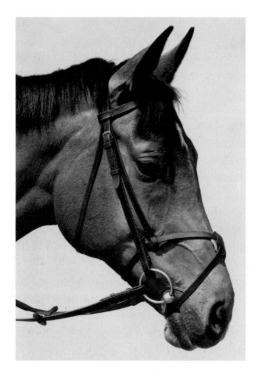

Fig. 5.6 Grakle noseband.

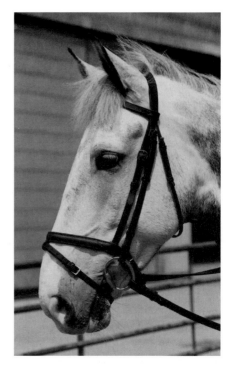

Fig. 5.7 Flash noseband.

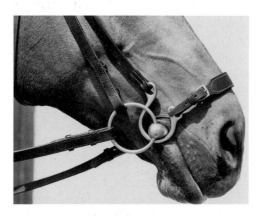

Fig. 5.8 Kineton noseband.

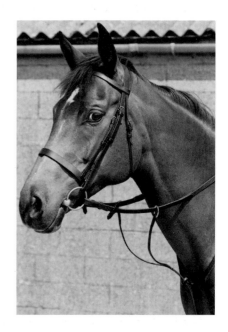

Fig. 5.9 Running martingale.

Europe and elsewhere in the world. However, if misused they can cause accidents and so must only be used properly by those trained and skilled in their use.

Standing martingale
The standing martingale acts downwards on the horse's nose when the horse lifts its head beyond the point of control. The martingale should be adjusted so that it does not interfere with the horse when it is carrying its head in an acceptable fashion, nor should it tie the horse down and prevent it jumping spread fences effectively. Some prefer to use the standing martingale to the running martingale as it does not interfere with the rein contact, particularly important with young horses. When standing in a relaxed position the martingale should be able to be pushed up into the horse's gullet.

Running martingale (Fig. 5.9)
The running martingale has the reins passing through the rings of the martingale thus acting to help keep the pressure on the bars of the horse's mouth when its head is raised. Correctly fitted the martingale should only come into play when the horse raises its head above a permitted level. Some horses resent the restriction of a running martingale. Stops must always be fitted to the reins when using a running martingale.

Market Harborough (Fig. 5.10)
The Market Harborough has a normal martingale body which splits in two, passes through the bit rings and fastens onto the reins. The action is to exert a strong downward pull on the bit when the horse throws its head up.

Draw reins
Sometimes referred to as running reins, the draw rein starts at the girth, passes through the front legs, through the bit rings and thus to the hand. The rein passes from the inside to the outside of the bit ring. Draw reins should be used with a normal rein placed above the draw rein. The draw rein may also be fitted so that it runs from the girth straps of the saddle, through the bit rings and back to the rider's hands.

Draw reins are useful for corrective training and can be used to prevent a fault occurring, not to establish a false tempo or outline. For example, if a horse persistently came above the bit in the canter transition, draw reins could be used to prevent this happening. Once the lesson has been learned the draw reins should be removed. Draw reins are also useful when doing

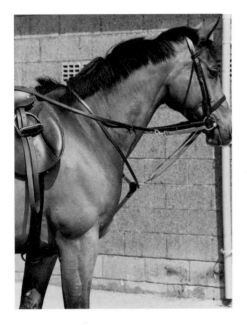

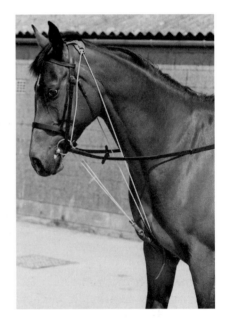

Fig. 5.10 Market Harborough martingale.   *Fig. 5.11* De Gogue.

fast work as they can help contain a strong horse and keep it round and encourage correct muscle development.

Chambon
The Chambon runs from the girth, between the horse's front legs, to the poll and then down to the bit to put pressure on the poll and induce lowered head carriage and a long, low outline. This encourages the correct muscle development and large, loose steps. It is only used on the lunge with a mild snaffle bit. Lungeing in a Chambon prior to ridden work can help relax a tense horse. The Chambon can only be effective if the horse accepts its action and responds correctly. This is achieved by first introducing the Chambon so that it does not affect the horse and gradually adjusting it a little every day. It should not be fitted tightly to fix the horse in a low outline. Horses with long necks or low set necks may be able to stretch down without influencing their backs; the Chambon is not effective for these horses.

De Gogue (Fig. 5.11)
The De Gogue is more advanced than the Chambon and can be used for ridden work as well as on the lunge. On the lunge the De Gogue has a strap running from the martingale body, (the part that runs between the horse's

legs before it joins the neckstrap) or saddle D, up one side of the face to the poll, to the bit and back to the martingale or saddle D, forming a triangle. For riding, instead of passing from the bit back to a fixed position, a rein is attached to the bit.

Side reins

Side reins can help in establishing a correct secure outline and good balance when working the horse on the lunge. Their main aim is to encourage the horse to reach down and seek contact with the bit. Reaching down will help extend the back and stretch the top of the neck. Side reins will also encourage the horse to step under and raise its back.

Side reins can be plain or have either elastic or rubber inserts to allow 'give'. They are fitted from the saddle or roller to the bit rings or cavesson. The fitting to the saddle or roller can be high or low but should not be lower than the point of the shoulder. Where they are fitted will be determined by the horse's conformation, its response to the side reins and what the trainer is hoping to achieve. If the horse has a poorly set neck the side reins are likely to be lower.

The length of the side reins is important and should be adjusted according to the age and experience of the horse, the trainer's objectives, the demands being imposed on the horse and the gait the horse is working in. The reins are the correct length if the horse is moving freely forward without restriction and at the same time using its back and hindquarters. Side reins will need to be longer in walk and canter than in trot. If the side reins are overshortened in an attempt to impose a posture on the horse the horse's paces will suffer.

Running side reins

Running side reins are an alternative to fixed side reins and offer greater freedom. Two reins, longer than fixed side reins, are fitted so that they pass from the roller to and through the bit rings and back to the roller. Running side reins can also be fitted as one long rein coming from one side of the roller, through the bit ring, over the poll, through the other bit ring and back the roller.

PART II

TRAINING THE RIDER FOR SHOW JUMPING AND CROSS-COUNTRY

6 Teaching the Inexperienced Rider

The aim of this chapter is to introduce the concept of the balanced jumping seat. Before attempting to teach the less experienced rider to jump, the correct seat must be established as it is the basic prerequisite for effective riding. The trainer's aim is to help the rider achieve a balanced independent seat without tension or stiffness. There are in effect three principal seat positions:

- dressage
- light
- jumping.

The dressage seat is the basic seat while the light seat allows the rider to change quickly to the dressage seat or the jumping seat. The light seat is useful for schooling jumpers on the flat and for hacking out as it combines security with lightness, allowing the rider to stay in balance and still be light on the horse's back. The stirrups are shorter and the rider leans the upper body slightly forward to lessen the pressure of the seat bones on the saddle. More of the rider's weight is carried by the thighs and knees with the joints of the hip, knee and ankle acting as springs to absorb the horse's movement. The seat does not leave the saddle and the lower legs stay stable, making the seat balanced and independent.

The balanced jumping seat (Figs 6.1 and 6.2)

The same basic principles apply to both riding on the flat and over fences. However, when the horse is jumping the centre of balance moves forward and the rider will need to adapt his or her position. The purpose of the jumping seat is to give freedom to the horse's back and to enable the rider to follow all changes in the horse's balance while still being able to influence the horse. In order to accommodate the horse's jump the stirrups will need

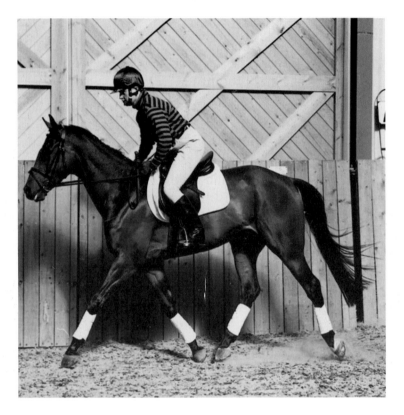

Fig. 6.1 The balanced jumping seat in trot.

to be shorter and the weight will need to be just out of the saddle. Between the fences the rider should adopt the light seat with the bottom near to the saddle and the security coming from a strong lower leg (Fig. 6.3). This position is emphasised during cross-country riding when the horse will have to cross varied terrain and does not want to be hindered by the rider's weight banging about on its back.

The rider's leg should remain firm and steady, the lower leg being by the girth and contributing a soft or strong forward influence on the horse. The leg should be ready to be strong if the need arises. The hip, knee and ankle joints must be flexible; the ability to stay in balance depends on the rider's ability to open and close the hip joint when necessary. If the jumping rider relies too much on the seat, tending to sit upright and drive the horse into the fence, then he or she will have to throw him or herself forward when the horse takes off in order to avoid being left behind. This

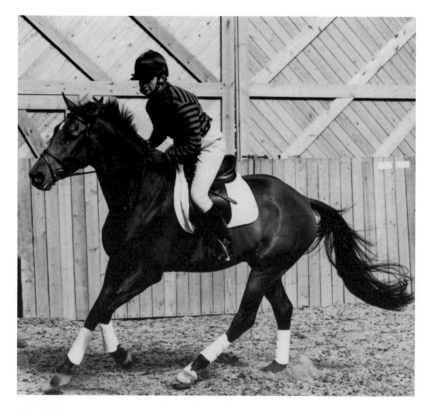

Fig. 6.2 The balanced jumping seat in canter.

can make the horse dive at the fence and possibly result in an unbalanced landing.

It is beneficial if the rider can keep the upper body as still as possible during the approach, over the fence and when riding away from the fence. If the upper body can be kept an angle of about 45° with the weight well down into the heels and a light seat, the rider need only offer the hand forward over the fence to give the horse sufficient freedom to make a good jump. The rider should be able to move the upper body forward fluently from the hips when necessary. Between the fences the hands should be quiet and steady so that the horse has to canter into the contact. The shoulder, elbow and wrist joints must be relaxed so that the rider's movements are not transmitted to the hands. The hands should be independent of the seat. Over the fence the rein can be offered either by the 'crest release' (Fig. 6.4) or by reaching down and forward on each side of the neck (Figs 6.5 and 6.6). The crest release

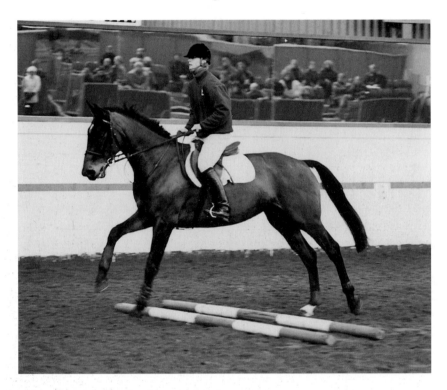

Fig. 6.3 A light balanced seat with a secure lower leg.

helps prevent the rider getting in front of the movement and avoids the rider's shoulders being lowered too much, which can cause the lower leg to slide back as the rider pivots on the knee.

If novice riders are taught to ride with slightly shorter stirrups so that they can adopt a light balanced seat and follow their horses' movements, they will progress to riding over small fences more easily. A jumping or general purpose saddle should be used as the knee roll will help to keep the knee steady. The foot may be pushed slightly further into the stirrup to help the lower leg stay firm.

Strengthening the position

The three main points of contact with the horse are the seat, the knee and the heel. Different muscles are used in this position compared with the dressage seat and novice riders will lack strength and tire easily. A useful

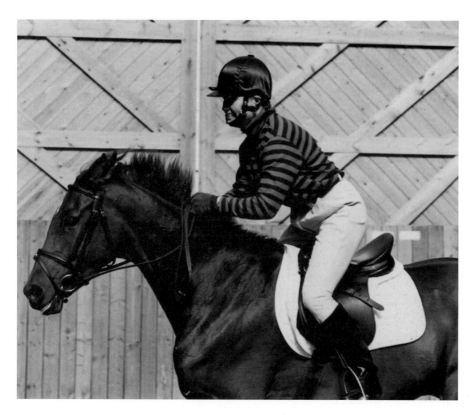

Fig. 6.4 Practising the crest release.

way to develop the rider's strength and balance is to practise riding in a 'two point position'. Here the rider does not put any weight on the seat, transferring all the weight to the stirrup (Fig. 6.7). This helps strengthen the effectiveness of the lower leg and establish a secure, independent position. Until the rider is able to maintain this balanced position in trot and canter he or she is unlikely to be able to stay in balance over a fence and will need to rely on the rein. If during this exercise the rider falls forward onto the horse's neck, the lower leg needs to be moved up to the girth, underneath the rider, for support. If the rider falls back into the saddle, the lower legs will have shot too far forward. The novice rider should be encouraged to hack out with jumping length stirrups, taking up the two point position up and down hill to further strengthen the leg position.

Transitions, both up and down, can also be made in the two point position. This will test whether the rider can stay in balance and also if the horse will

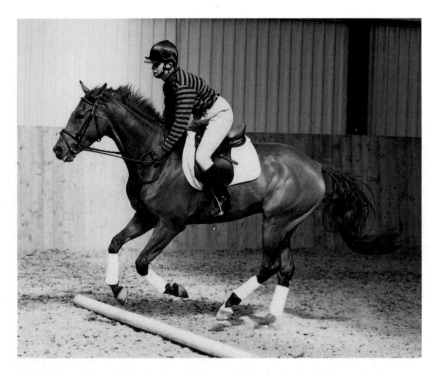

Fig. 6.5 Practising the release down and forward either side of the neck over a pole.

go off the leg without the use of the seat. Many riders find it necessary to sit in the saddle and drive the horse into canter, for example, rather than just using the leg.

The lightness of the seat can be varied depending on what is required and this can also be practised by the novice rider. When the stride is free and open the seat should barely brush the saddle. However, when executing a tight turn the rider brings back the shoulders and the seat comes close to the saddle; this collects the horse's stride and brings the centre of balance back. The rider can practise this until the horse will shorten the stride by the rider merely moving his or her body weight, without having to pull on the reins at all. Should the horse back off excessively from a fence the rider can still call upon the seat as a driving aid to help negotiate the fence.

The cross-country position (Fig. 6.8)

The jumping position is further exaggerated when riding cross-country; the stirrups are shortened again to close up the angles between the hips, knees

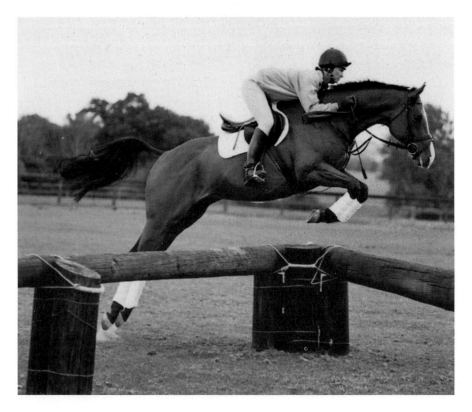

Fig. 6.6 The rein release cross-country.

and ankles. This in turn pushes the seat further to the back of the saddle and pulls the knees up further forward; a cross-country saddle must have forward cut flaps and a large enough seat. As before, the seat is lightened and brought out of the saddle, supported by a strong lower leg with the weight in the heels. The security of the lower leg is vital for safe cross-country riding. The lower leg must stay in position to counterbalance the upper body which will move around considerably during the course of a cross-country round. The aim is to ride with a secure, balanced and independent seat so that the rider can stay in balance with the horse on the approach, in the air, on landing and during the getaway. When cantering downhill the lower leg can be allowed a little more forward with the shoulders up and back. When cantering uphill the lower leg must not be allowed to slip back with the upper body too far forward.

Between the fences the weight should be out of the saddle with the upper body inclined slightly forward and the lower leg still. The shoulders, head

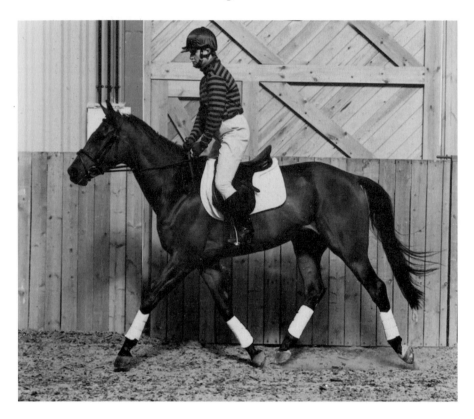

Fig. 6.7 Varying the seat in trot to improve strength and balance.

and neck should be kept up, with the hands close to the horse's neck, just in front of the withers. On the approach to the fence the rider should sit up and keep the shoulders up; the rider may sit lightly on or above the saddle with the lower leg in contact with the horse and ready to be used strongly if necessary. The hands should be low and quiet and ready to correct the horse if it wavers off line.

Overcoming fear

Many novice riders will be anxious about jumping. Fear can stem from many sources, for example the fear of the pain caused by falling off or simply from severe discomfort experienced when riding. These fears need to be discovered and allayed as far as possible. The fear of a fall can be helped by using

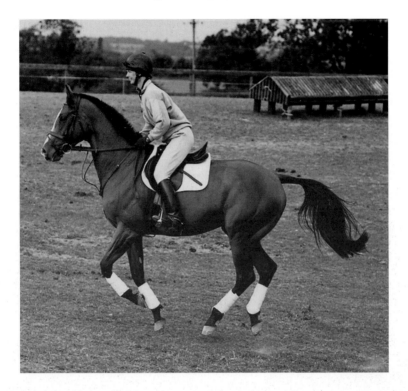

Fig. 6.8 The cross-country position.

sufficient explanation and direction throughout every stage of the learning process and by adhering to sound, safe teaching practice.

Fear of failure or ridicule is very significant. As a teacher remember the difficulties you encountered when last mastering a new skill; always try to set achievable goals and never be sarcastic or short tempered. The teacher must be particularly careful when teaching groups that the competitive tendency of the participants is kept under control so that no one is made to feel inferior.

The theory of jumping

Novice riders should be encouraged to seek in their horses and themselves:

- rhythm
- impulsion

- feel
- balance
- confidence
- timing
- control.

The track

The route that the rider takes before, between and after the fence will affect the way the horse is presented to the fence and whether the horse can successfully negotiate the fence. Many novice riders are so concerned about getting over the jump that they forget about getting to the fence, the horse is badly presented and stops or makes an uncomfortable jump. If the novice rider has steering problems before or after the fence, Bloks or poles can be strategically placed so that the rider has to steer around or between them before and after the fence (Fig. 6.9). Even from very early lessons the trainer

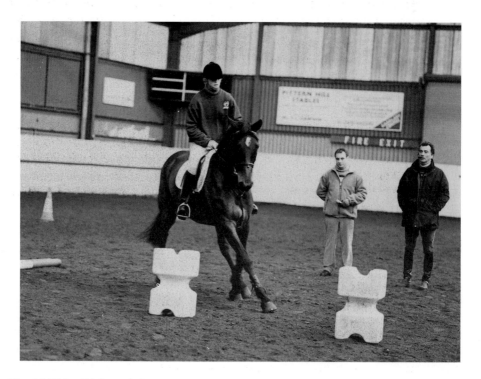

Fig. 6.9 Using Bloks to help to turn to the fence.

must emphasise the importance of the route taken to the fence. The trainer must also teach the rider how to start and finish the exercise, in other words how to prepare the horse for the task, especially in a class lesson situation where the horse may have been standing still for some time. On completing the exercise the horse must not be allowed to dive back to its companions but should make correct downwards transitions in good style. If these good habits are instilled in the novice rider they will become second nature.

The approach

During the turn to the fence the rider keeps an eye on the fence so that he or she can trace the track correctly. The turn can be used to the rider's advantage, improving the horse's balance, engaging the hocks and getting the horse off its forehand. However, the turn is often neglected resulting in the horse arriving at the fence out of balance and with little impulsion. The rider must endeavour to make a good job of the turn and wait until the horse has completed the turn before riding forward to the fence. If the rider has not managed to get the horse all the way round the turn its quarters will be on a different track to the forehand so that when the rider rides forward to the fence the horse will not be able to transmit the impulsion effectively.

On the approach to the fence the rider should look up and over the fence to the next obstacle. This prevents the rider looking down and getting 'stuck' in the ground, inviting the horse to stop or knock down the fence. The rider must ensure that the rhythm, impulsion and balance of the trot or canter are of good quality. Maintaining a light balanced seat the rider should have supple hips, flat level shoulders, elastic arms and the hands should be fairly close together, low and close to the horse's neck.

The last three strides

During the last three strides the rider should remain in the balanced seat, only allowing the seat to come into the saddle and drive the horse if the horse backs off the fence. The horse must be allowed to concentrate on negotiating the fence. The rider's hands should maintain the contact, moving towards the horse's mouth as the horse's head and neck lower for the take-off. The rider should not 'throw' the reins at the horse in the last stride; this is disconcerting for the horse and the rider may then have to snatch the rein back on landing. Novice riders who lack confidence and worry about not being able to see a stride, may 'freeze' during the last three strides. Their confidence can be built up using a placing fence or small fences at related distances.

The take-off

The rider must wait for the horse to jump the fence, not 'going before the horse' or 'getting in front of the movement'. The rider should keep a steady contact with the leg and reins, allowing the horse to use its head and neck freely (Fig. 6.10). The upper body should be kept as still as possible; the rider need only offer the hand forward over the fence to give the horse sufficient freedom to make a good jump. It may be helpful for the rider to think of the horse's withers coming up to meet the rider and to allow the hand forward so that the amount of release is determined by how much the horse wants to use its head and neck. If the rider just thinks of folding the upper body, the hands tend to get stuck on the withers. The rider should be able to move the

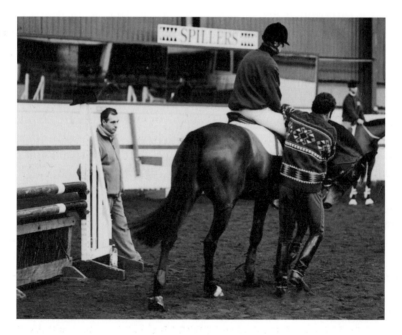

Fig. 6.10 Helping the rider to understand the rein contact.

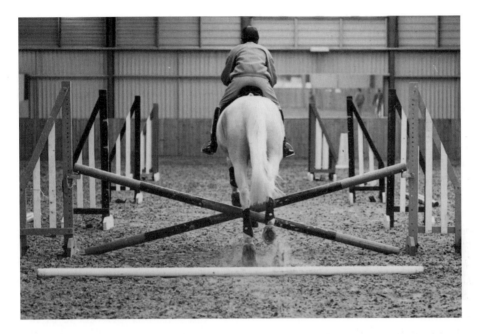

Fig. 6.11 The importance of straightness.

upper body forward fluently from the hips when necessary. The rider should look ahead along the track he or she intends to follow or to the next fence while remaining straight (Fig. 6.11).

The landing

The rider's contact and influences should stay the same, with the upper body at the same angle of 45°, staying in balance with the horse. If necessary the rider can adopt a slightly more upright position in order to steady the pace, improve the impulsion, re-establish the balance or to make a turn or downward transition.

The first lessons

Teaching a novice adult in a riding school is in many ways easier than teaching someone who has gone out and bought themselves a horse that may not be suitable. The riding school, however, must ensure that the horse selected for the client is a suitable size and shape and familiar with the level of work demanded. The saddle must also fit the client, with leathers and irons a proper fit.

Throughout the early lessons demonstration is a useful aid to learning, as is having a valid reason for teaching something a certain way. Thus the novice should not just be told to hold the reins in a certain way or to adopt a particular position in the saddle; the teacher should also explain why these things are done that way. At each stage check that the riders have fully understood what has been said and encourage them to tell you how they are feeling as the lesson progresses. Remember throughout that riders must not be given too much to think about at once; they need to be able to focus on one target at a time. Each stage should be clearly explained and taught in easily assimilated chunks.

At this stage it is probably a good idea to begin to introduce the 'what if' scenarios. What if the horse does not go forward from the leg, what if the horse does not respond to a turning aid, what if the horse fails to stop when asked, what if the horse spooks at the fence? If the teacher suggests ideas to the riders as to how they should try to react, it may prove useful in an emergency.

The golden rules for teaching novice riders are:

- The rider should progress at the speed at which he or she feels confident.
- Safety and good practice must be top of the teacher's list of priorities.
- The teacher must be enthusiastic.
- Each pupil must feel that he or she is important.
- The novice rider should never be pushed or overfaced.
- For many adult learners the social aspect of riding is important; if they want to discuss their children, home, clothes or politics, the teacher should show lively and responsive interest.

Remember that beginner riders will be using different muscles which are not fit; it is sometimes difficult for the regular rider to remember how quickly these unfit muscles tire and become sore. The teacher must be aware of this and plan the lesson accordingly.

Common rider faults

The trainer needs to not only recognise the fault but also assess the cause of the fault. Frequently faults arise because riders are anxious about jumping.

If this is so, merely telling these riders to correct their positions will be ineffective. Riders need to be given confidence before they can concentrate on what their bodies are doing in the spilt second over a fence.

Stirrup leathers too long or short
If the leathers are too long the rider's position will be weak and ineffective, and he or she will also find it hard to stay in balance. However, the trainer must resist the temptation to shorten the leathers too dramatically as many novice riders find riding short not only painful but also frightening. Time should be spent working on the flat in the balanced seat to build up the rider's strength, confidence and balance. If the leathers are too short the rider will be insecure and inclined to get in front of the horse's movement.

Reins too long or short
Most novice riders are concerned about 'getting left behind' and jabbing the horse in the mouth. This can tend to make them ride with long reins in an attempt to give the horse freedom of the head and neck. In fact it has just the wrong effect; the rider becomes out of balance, gets behind the movement and the jump is uncomfortable for both horse and rider. If the reins are too short the rider tends to get pulled forward as the horse approaches the fence, again getting out of balance. Some riders, in an attempt to help the horse and give it freedom of its head and neck, drop the contact on the last stride and over the fence. This can be disturbing for the horse and it may stop or make an unbalanced jump. On landing, the rider has to snatch up the reins to regain the contact, again unbalancing the horse.

Looking down
Many experienced riders are guilty of looking down on the approach to the fence and over the fence. The trainer must encourage the rider to look up and beyond the fence, to the track he or she is to follow on landing, or the next fence, or even a spot on the horizon.

Too much movement over the fence
The rider's hands, lower legs or upper body may move too much over the fence, often due to lack of security and confidence. Riders should practise the balanced seat in trot and canter and through transitions until they are strong and secure. A neck strap is an essential piece of equipment for the novice rider.

'Firing' the horse at the fence

The over-keen rider or the rider who lacks the confidence to 'wait for the fence to come to him or her', may sit in the saddle and press the horse to the fence in the last few strides. This usually results in the horse gathering speed and flattening over the fence. The trainer must establish why the rider is riding like this and use appropriate exercises to help, such as small fences at related distances.

Rider anatomy

In the dressage seat the weight of the rider's body rests on the lower edges of the two hip bones. The angle of the pelvis and the curves of the spinal column adapt and they adopt this sitting position so that the hip bones assume a more upright position and the hollow in the small of the back virtually disappears, straightening the spine. The rider's head is poised over the centre of the hip joints creating an upright balanced seat. When the rider adopts a light seat the rider tilts the pelvis forward to balance and carry the weight down into the knees and heels.

The thigh bone or femur is the longest bone in the body. The length and strength of the thigh helps the rider to stay in balance and to give aids to the horse. The rider with a short thigh will find it more difficult to stay in balance.

The influence of the rider when jumping (Fig. 6.12)

The rider can all too easily hamper the horse, preventing it from jumping correctly and effectively. The horse should jump the same way under saddle as it does loose.

On approaching the fence it is the rider's task to check the impulsion and to steer the horse towards the middle of the fence. However, all adjustments must be made without unsettling the horse. On no account should the hands pull backwards – the horse must be free to stretch its head and neck as much as it wants to. As the horse takes off it is important that the rider follows the movement; one common fault is that the rider, worried of being left behind, comes too far forward, interfering with the horse's rhythm. Over the fence riders should aim to keep their upper body nearly parallel with the horse's back and neck and their lower legs straight down. They should bend forward as much as is necessary to follow the horse's movements. Enthusiastic riders

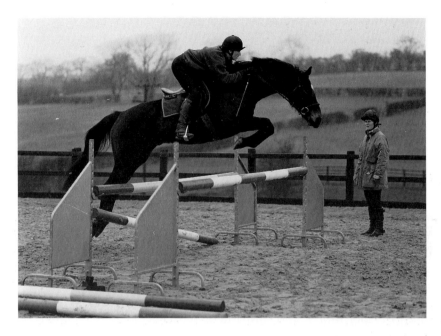

Fig. 6.12 The rider's position enables the young horse to jump a spread fence with confidence.

must take care that they do not get in front of the horse – extravagant stretching of the arms towards the horse's ears disturbs its balance. Landing is difficult for the horse; the rider can help by sitting lightly and giving with the hands and arms to allow the horse to regain its balance after the fence. The first canter stride is decided by the horse's own impulsion; it is only at the second stride that the rider can start to influence the horse without disturbing the rhythm.

Summary

- Overall aim: to help the rider achieve a balanced independent seat without tension or stiffness.
- By developing:
    self awareness
    discipline
    feel for the horse

     confidence

     increasing knowledge.

- Method

     explanation of the three principal seat positions

     varying the seat to develop strength and balance

     explanation of the phases of the jump

     the rider should progress at the speed at which he or she feels
       confident

     safety and good practice must be top of the teacher's list of priorities

     the teacher must be enthusiastic

     each pupil must feel that he or she is important

     the novice rider should never be pushed or over-faced.

- The tools of the trade

     horse – must be suitable

     equipment – the right saddle

               videos or guinea pigs for demonstration and explanation.

- Likely problems

     lack of rider fitness and suppleness

     rider losing balance

     lack of confidence.

7 Developing the Rider's Skill

After the basic skills described in the previous chapter have been established the goal is to develop the rider's ability to maintain the quality of the work at all times. The teacher needs to make sure that the rider takes some responsibility for his or her own discipline. The teacher must ensure that the rider continues to develop his or her eye and remain open-minded in the quest for further knowledge. Whilst there are certain guidelines that the teacher should not deviate from, these ideals must allow for the idiosyncrasies of both horse and rider.

The qualities of the jumping teacher

There are no differences in the qualities required to be a successful trainer of jumping as opposed to riding on the flat. The most difficult thing any teacher of riding has to do is to look at the whole picture as there is a huge amount to observe in one moment. As the horse and rider progress it requires increasing skill to do this. At first the teacher may have to focus on the main theme of the lesson, which is easily observable, before being able to pick up the subtleties of the wider view. Thus at first the teacher may concentrate on the position of the rider's lower leg, the smoothness and success of the jump or whether the rider is in balance. Once the teacher is comfortable with this he or she can move on to look at the balance and impulsion of the horse before progressing to look at the bascule, the position of the horse's forehand and hindquarters. In other words, teachers should look at one thing at a time until they develop their eye. This structured approach to training will also benefit the rider.

The theme of the present lesson may be 'the rider's lower leg' (Fig. 7.1). In order to be able to concentrate on this aspect the horse must perform relatively smoothly, allowing the rider to become really secure. To obtain a smooth jump the teacher may have to help the rider present the horse to the fence better. The teacher must also pay detailed attention to the building

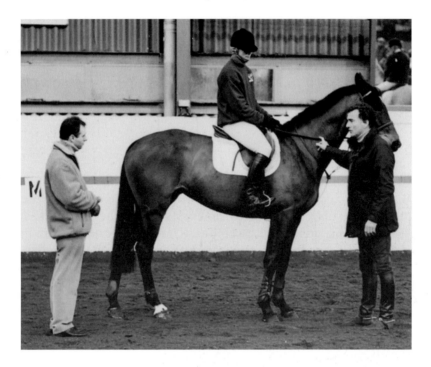

Fig. 7.1 The correct lower leg.

and siting of the fences. If these details are not correct it will be more difficult for the rider to get the smooth jump necessary before the teacher can start to concentrate on the lower leg. The developing trainer may not be able to observe the shape the horse makes over the fence and the technique of its limbs as well as all the foregoing requirements.

The schoolmaster horse (Fig. 7.2)

In order to achieve our goals with relative ease it is essential to be equipped with a suitable horse or pony and a saddle that fits both horse and rider.

What makes an ideal schoolmaster?

- First and foremost the horse must be genuine and reliable in its attitude to jumping. If unsure whether or not the horse is going to jump, the nervous rider tends to ride defensively while the more confident rider will tend to ride aggressively, neither of which are ideal attitudes to jumping.

- Ideally the horse should make a smooth jump with some bascule. However, excessive bascule makes it hard for the developing rider to stay in balance.
- It is quite reasonable for the horse to be keen to get to the fence, so long as it remains under control. Its head carriage should be stable, it may be a little too high or too low, but providing it is not unstable this is not detrimental in the schoolmaster.

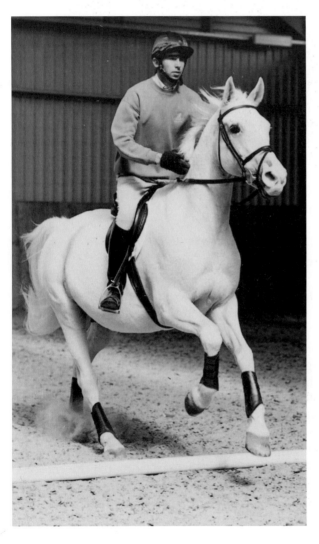

Fig. 7.2 The ideal schoolmaster horse.

- Alternatively it does not matter if the horse is a little lazy provided that it does not grind to a halt when it gets to the fence.

The teacher should equip the horse for the maximum benefit of both horse and rider. A snaffle with no martingale may be the 'ideal'; however, this may not be possible as schoolmasters are often older horses that have competed in the past and are used to other forms of restraint.

Novice rider, novice horse

Many riders yearn to buy a young horse so that they can learn and grow together, just as children are bought a puppy to grow up with. However, if mistakes are made training a puppy all that will probably happen is that it develops a few endearing bad habits, such as jumping on the furniture. If mistakes are made in the training of a young horse the consequences are likely to be much more serious. The horse may start to jump badly, for example with a hollow back, which increase the chance of it developing physical problems. It may then start to refuse to jump and eventually become totally nappy. For these reasons alone novice riders should be urged to work with experienced horses until the teacher feels that they are sufficiently skilled to train a horse themselves.

Matching horse and rider

The next vital role for the teacher is to match horse and rider for maximum benefit. The key factors to take into account here include:

- Rider enjoyment – one of the teacher's main priorities must be that the rider enjoys developing his or her skills; thus the horse's personality should suit that particular rider. If the teacher has worked with the rider before, the teacher will know whether the rider is more at ease with a keen horse or something rather steadier. If it is the rider's first lesson the teacher must talk to the pupil to find out as much as possible and so that the rider feels that the lesson is a joint venture.
- Size and type – the size and type of the horse must match the rider. At this stage tall riders should not be mounted on small horses and short riders should not be matched with large horses. Equally the horse must be able to carry the rider's weight with ease.

Having decided on these two vital factors and providing that the horse meets the other schoolmaster requirements, the teacher should start the lesson with a happy, confident combination.

Buying a horse for a novice rider

Helping a client to buy a horse is more problematic than matching horse and rider for a lesson. It is a good idea to sit down with the client and make a list of priorities. For example, the client is a keen young man in his mid-twenties, 182 cm (6 ft) tall and weighing 70 kg (11 stone) who eventually would like to hunt and team chase. However, at this stage he only has basic jumping skills, confidently jumping 2 ft 6 in (0.7 m). He is to keep the horse at livery with the teacher.

- Mares – some riders are prejudiced against mares. If the teacher works well with mares and the client is not an aggressive rider, keeping an open mind about buying a mare will certainly increase the opportunities to buy.
- Size – a client of this height would ideally buy a 16 hh (166 cm) to 16.2 hh (169 cm) middleweight horse.
- Age – ideally the horse will be experienced and therefore is likely to be a minimum of eight years old. As the rider's skill and ambition develop it is possible that he may want to sell the horse; thus it may be wise to have a maximum age of 12 years old.
- Experience – the horse should have been hunting, show jumped to Newcomers level and hunter trialled or evented. The teacher should look for this wide range of experience so that he or she can follow the ideal training philosophy, which is that the rider should become multi-skilled even if the ultimate desire is only to hunt and team chase.
- Type – ideally the horse will be half or three-quarter bred with an amicable temperament. The breeding is not crucial, but a thoroughbred is unlikely to be suitable as most tend to be quite sharp to ride. All teachers will have had experience of a range of breeds and this experience may indicate that a certain breed of horse may not suit the temperament of the rider.
- Price – a horse is worth what somebody is prepared to pay for it. For this client an experienced schoolmaster is worth more than a four-year-old with potential. Remember that the purchase price is just the beginning of the cost and a bad horse costs as much to keep as a good one. Generally

the client should be prepared to spend as much as he or she can afford and not look for a bargain; there is nearly always a catch.

It is vital that the inexperienced purchaser has help and advice when buying a horse, preferably from his or her own teacher. Failing that, the client could be sent to a reputable dealer, from whom the teacher has previously bought horses and whom the teacher trusts to look after the client. Problems can arise if the client 'falls in love' with a horse which does not match up to all the requirements outlined. The teacher must weigh up the situation, evaluating the advantages and disadvantages of the horse. Above all the client should be discouraged from buying a young, inexperienced horse – it rarely makes for a happy, successful partnership.

The rider is now equipped with a suitable horse and lessons can begin. As with any sport how often the rider practises will determine to some extent the speed at which progress is made.

Developing rider technique

When the stage of developing rider technique is reached riders are often keen to progress quickly to larger fences. The teacher must try to convince them that developing style and technique over smaller fences will, in the long run, enable them to reach their ultimate goal more quickly. The rider must understand that technique is vital to success.

In other sports, such as tennis, running, boxing and swimming, the top athletes take time to study and analyse their technique with their trainers. They appreciate that even tiny weaknesses can make the difference between winning and losing. The film 'Chariots of Fire' demonstrates that even in 1923 coaches were concerned with improving performance by mere seconds. The horses and riders we teach will perform at their best if they are trained to maximise their potential by adhering to the ideals of the time. It is difficult to place in order of priority the skills the teacher should develop in the rider. They include balance, rhythm, transitions and turning.

Balance
Perhaps the major skill to develop is that of the rider keeping the horse balanced, especially in canter. In other words, as far as possible the weight of the horse and that of the rider should be spread over all four legs in such a way as to enable the horse to use itself with optimum ease and efficiency.

Loss of balance is frequently characterised by the horse falling on to its forehand which feels as if it is going downhill; the rider must learn to recognise when this happens. It is the teacher's job to observe the moment and alert the rider so that the rider can feel the moment and then adjust the horse accordingly. The adjustment may be a half halt or an alteration to rider position, particularly if the rider has become in front of the movement. Other signs of loss of balance include the horse falling either in or out through the shoulders, especially on corners and circles, when the horse may either drift to the inside or fail to turn accurately.

Rhythm

If the tempo, i.e. the speed of the rhythm, is wrong for the particular exercise that is being carried out the horse will tend to lose its balance. Rhythm and balance are inextricably linked and developing the rider's awareness of rhythm, tempo and balance is vital to the rider's progress. Initially exercises without fences, especially outside, should be used to help the rider discover the feel of the horse's rhythm, tempo and balance. Subsequently experimental tempo work with poles (Fig. 7.3) and fences can be introduced. A useful exercise involves the rider counting the strides in canter, simply 1, 2, 3, 4 and so on. The teacher can introduce a pole on the ground and the rider will find that the pole fits somewhere into the rhythm, for example:

1	2	3	4	5	6	7	8	9	10 etc.
				pole				pole	

Once a single pole can be negotiated in rhythm then a series of poles can be introduced, up to a total of six poles if room and material allows (Fig. 7.4). Initially three poles can be used 2.4 m (8–9 ft) apart, but this distance should be altered to accommodate the horse's natural rhythm and stride length. At this stage the aim is for the rider to become aware of the ease of the rhythm and develop a feel for a contained, active and round canter stride. During this exercise the rider should remain in a light position with the seat close to the saddle but not resting in it. The stirrups should be at a length that allows this position to be maintained and the rein contact should be kept with the hands on either side of the neck. If the rider adopts this position there should be no need to change the position either over the poles or round the arena. The only time the rider would need to alter the position is if the horse loses the balance, for example if the horse tries to hurry onto its forehand the rider should come a little more upright with his or her shoulders, or if the horse becomes sluggish the rider may need to use his or her legs vigorously. It

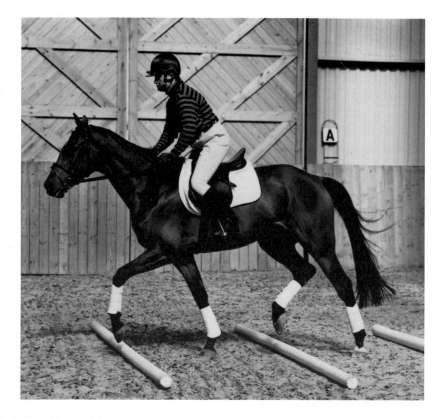

Fig. 7.3 Trotting poles.

should not, however, be necessary to drive with the seat. Watch a National Hunt jockey. He does not use his seat but relies on his legs and this skill should be developed with the jumping rider. Later, in competition when under pressure the rider may have to resort to all sorts of means if the situation demands it, but when training try to remain classical.

Even at this stage the rider must be encouraged to look ahead and not down at the pole. The rider must learn to trust the horse to work things out for itself. This does not mean that the rider never looks at the pole or the fence, but simply that he or she does not focus on it to the exclusion of all else, which tends to make the rider collapse his or her position and lose control.

Once the rider is established cantering over poles set at the ideal distance then the stride can be lengthened and shortened to heighten the rider's experience and feel. Eventually the rider will know when the horse feels at its most comfortable. In later exercises the rider will canter over a series of poles on the way to a fence and through a series of fences; thus the rider must be confident to canter over poles on the flat. The initial exercise is best introduced on a straight line, but later it can be ridden on a curve, which gives an added choice of distances. However, the rider must be able to ride the horse on an accurate circle before introducing the ground poles.

Transitions

The trainer needs to teach the rider to be able to move up and down the 'gear box' without the horse becoming resistant to either the upward or downward aids and without the frame of the horse changing too much. Again the role of the teacher is vital in observing the horse's reaction to the aids and checking through questioning that the rider is able to feel the responses of the horse. The rider should be able to recognise, for example, when the horse has not responded immediately to a forward aid and develop an almost instinctive reaction to this. What form this reaction takes may vary from horse to horse, from a flick with the whip to a firmer leg aid. The

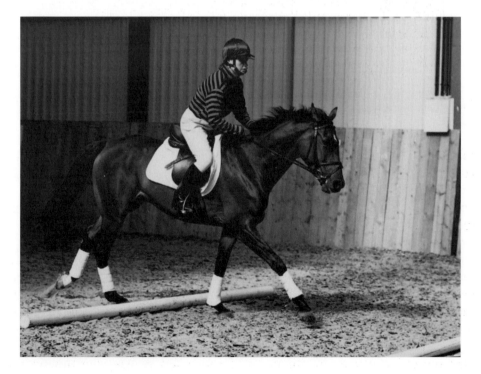

Fig. 7.4 A series of canter poles.

teacher and rider must experiment so that the rider can find out how reactions can vary.

Turning

The horse must respond willingly to the rider's turning aids, the main problem here being loss of the outside shoulder resulting in the horse falling to the inside and changing legs behind if the balance is lost.

  The teacher should start with simple exercises, for example riding an accurate 20 m circle. The exercises can then be built up and become more complex, for example using cones, Bloks and poles to map out a route for the rider to follow. This exercise is both useful and fun but the turns should never be so sharp that the horse cannot maintain the rhythm. The level of training of the horse and rider combination should be kept in mind as the exercises progress. If the rider cannot canter a 10 m circle in balance with a light seat, the exercise must not include a 10 m half-circle turn. If changes of canter lead are to be incorporated at this stage, they should be through trot and there should be plenty of room. The rider can practise until the change can be accomplished with no more than one or two strides in trot. The ideal is to have a rider who is able to canter a course through jump wings or Bloks before he or she actually embarks on jumping a course. This should start as

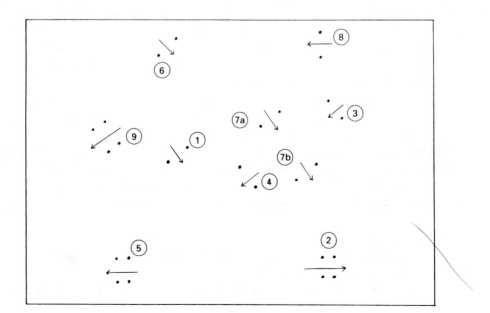

Fig. 7.5 Riding a line through a 'course' of Bloks.

a simple figure-of-eight and work up to a fairly complex course such as the one shown in Fig. 7.5. Although this course is complex it is flowing which helps the rider to develop manoeuvring skills.

If the lesson is on an artificial surface the teacher can draw a line for the pupils to follow, so that they learn right from the outset how to place the horse on a line and keep it there without it drifting. If the horse does drift the teacher must tell the riders and encourage them to feel the difference between the horse remaining straight or veering off a line. This skill will be useful to the riders later on as it will alert them to the fact that the horse is tending to run out at a fence and it will also help them plan and adhere to the most effective route in a jump-off. Often at this stage the trainer has to keep reminding the pupil of why it is important to be disciplined and to pay attention to detail.

Introducing jumping

Once the rider can maintain the balance, rhythm and tempo on the flat and over poles and ride a line through a course of wings, he or she has to learn to apply the same principles to jumping. The teacher should build a simple fence that will encourage the rider to maintain the balance, rhythm and tempo whilst still keeping the classical light seat. The rider should be encouraged to count the strides, but always upwards, i.e. 1, 2, 3, not 3, 2, 1, *go*. The latter encourages the rider to 'fire' the horse at the fence which is not in accord with our methodology. A suitable fence to start with would be an upright with a ground pole on both the take-off and landing side of the fence to allow the fence to be jumped off both reins. The fence would probably be 2 ft 9 in to 3 ft (0.8–0.9 m) high with the ground pole about 2 ft (0.6 m) away from the fence to give a take-off line.

The teacher should try to look at the overall picture of the rider and conscientiously correct positional faults. This will give the rider plenty of confidence and security as he or she progresses through the exercise. However, remember the golden rules of making corrections:

- One thing at a time.
- Do not distract riders as they approach the fence.
- Praise improvement, however slight.
- Use pupil-led self-evaluation as well as instructor-led learning, and encourage pupils to be positive in their evaluation.
- Encourage pupils to evaluate the horse as well as themselves.

- Always be prepared to discuss any correction made or, indeed, any situation that riders feel uncomfortable about.
- Encourage pupils to seek a solution to any problems that arise; do not just hand them the answer on a plate.

Jumping sequences (Figs 7.6–7.8)

When the pupil can arrive at the fence, jump and land in reasonable balance (not yet perhaps perfect balance), a second fence of the same height and construction can be introduced three strides away. A distance of about 42 ft (12.8 m) measured from jump wing to jump wing should be used. Initially a tape measure should be used until the trainer is completely confident in his or her ability to stride a distance accurately.

   Once again the rider should be encouraged to maintain the light seat throughout, thus reducing the need for excessive folding over the fence, which tends to unbalance both horse and rider, especially at the early stages of development (Fig. 7.9). The counting technique can be used once more to develop further the rider's awareness of rhythm. Watch out for the rider counting landing over the first fence as a stride; the rider must count the first

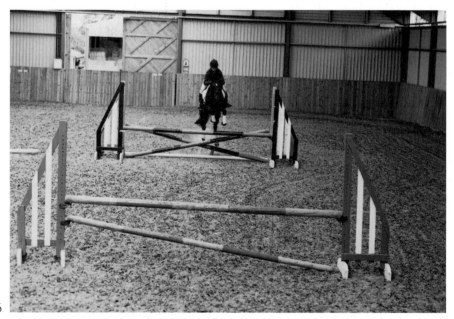

7.6

Figs 7.6–7.8 Introducing sequence jumping.

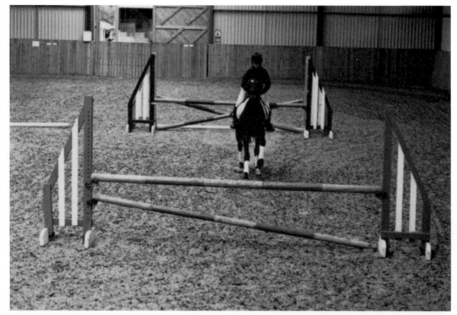

7.7

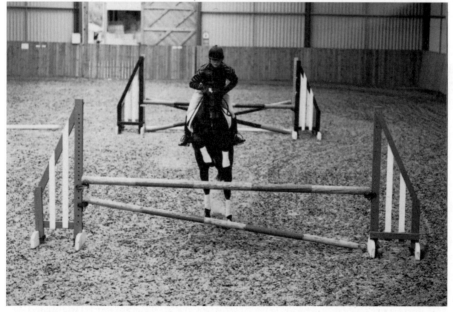

7.8

Figs 7.6–7.8 Introducing sequence jumping (cont.).

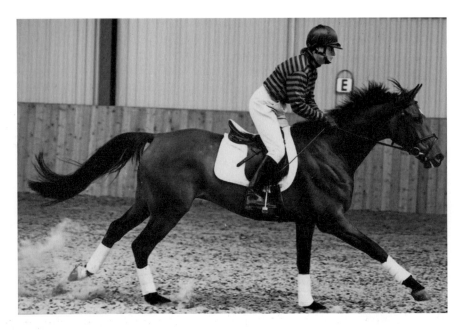

Fig. 7.9 The balanced seat between fences.

full stride after landing and will take off over the second fence as the third stride is completed.

Most riders find the introduction to sequence jumping easier if they are given time between the two fences, rather than progressing straight to a double. The trainer must carefully observe that the distance between the two fences is ideal for the horse and rider combination and alter the distance if necessary.

Jumping doubles

The rider can now be introduced to two stride (Fig. 7.10) and one stride doubles. In order to keep the rider confident and to avoid a drama should a mistake occur, it is wise to make the fences verticals with clear ground poles. The fences for these exercises do not need to be more than 2 ft 9 in (0.8 m) to 3 ft (0.9 m) and for two strides out of canter should be 33 ft (10 m) apart. The rider should be encouraged to remain in a light balanced seat between fences, simply allowing the horse to take as much rein as it wants without losing the contact.

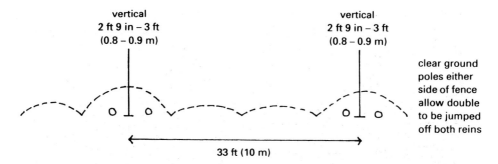

Fig. 7.10 Introducing a two-stride double.

Once again the rider should be asked for feedback:

- Did the horse have to stretch for the second element?
- Did it seem to have to 'put in a short one'?
- Was the horse in the correct rhythm and tempo?
- Was the horse 'in front of the leg', in other words was it willing to go forwards?

These questions should be asked before the distance between the two fences is altered; at this stage the teacher wants the rider to get the best possible feel over the fences. The rider is not yet ready to be asked to alter the horse's approach to and through the double; that arises later in the training regime. When the rider is confident and can stay in balance throughout the approach, jump, landing and getaway, a one stride double can be introduced. The construction and height of the fences should stay the same with a distance of 21 ft (6.4 m) between the two elements.

Riding a course

The next logical step is to link the fences together into a simple course. A figure-of-eight with one change of direction is sufficient at this stage. The fences should remain simple verticals with ground poles placed so that the turns are easy and flowing to encourage the rider to keep the horse in balance.

The teacher should focus on how the rider influences the horse in between the fences. One of the finest axioms of jumping is 'look after the canter and the jump will look after itself'. The late Caroline Bradley, one of the most stylish and successful show jumpers, was even heard to quote this and she practised the art of 'allowing the horse to do the jumping' to a high degree. To reach this stage with one rider having two lessons a week would probably take about 20 lessons, assuming that there are no setbacks and that the preliminary work has been completed successfully. The rider will not be perfect but will probably be ready to progress to the next stage which involves introducing different types of fences and grids.

Jumping spread fences (Fig. 7.11)

When introducing a spread fence it is often best to use it as the second jump of a three stride related distance. An ascending oxer is probably the easiest fence to start with, and should be about 2 ft 9 in (0.8 m) in front and 3 ft (0.9 m) at the back with a spread of 2 ft 9 in (0.8 m) to 3 ft (0.9 m). The front can be filled in with a drop pole supported with a cup. The whole fence must be built so that it can fall if hit hard.

When the rider is confident about the feel of a spread fence the type of fence can be varied to include a cross pole with a rail behind (Fig. 7.12) and a true parallel. The height and spread should stay the same. The rider will now begin to feel which of these fences is the easiest for him or her. Often the rider prefers to jump the spread fence shown in Fig. 7.12, but care must be taken that the cross is not too high or too low. If it is too high and the horse does not stay straight it will either have to jump very big or screw sideways to clear the fence. If the cross is too low the horse may dive over the fence rather than jump it in good style.

The rider can now be introduced to jumping a spread fence on its own, from canter. Again the rider should be encouraged to count the rhythm; over these small training fences it is not necessary for the rider to change the

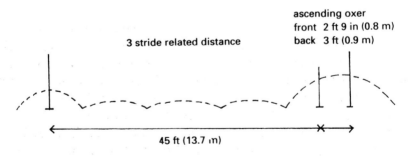

Fig. 7.11 Introducing spread fences: ascending oxer with drop pole.

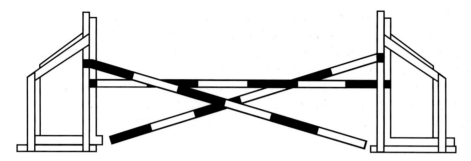

Fig. 7.12 Cross pole with a rail behind.

horse's tempo. Frequently the rider comes to the conclusion that it is easier to jump a spread than an upright and that the sensation is much more agreeable. As the rider progresses the three types of spread fence can be introduced in different circumstances. However, for novice riders and novice horses a spread coming out of a one stride double is not recommended, as there is less margin for error.

All of these exercises can be practised indoors or outside, on artificial surfaces or on grass. Indeed, using a variety of situations like this will now be very beneficial to the rider. If fillers are available and the horse is confident jumping them, these can occasionally be incorporated into the lesson. It is important that the fillers are not too high; a maximum height of 2 ft 6 in (0.7 m) is sufficient. This again is to reduce the risk factor with the novice rider. At each stage of the rider's learning process it is useful to ask the rider to ride the simple course again to check that all the main criteria are adhered to and are becoming increasingly confirmed.

Grid work

The time has now come to develop the rider's balance and co-ordination further by introducing grid work. Before this, however, the rider should be introduced to bounce fences (Fig. 7.13). To keep the rider's confidence the exercise should start in trot and be kept small. Using a cross pole to a vertical is ideal; the rider can ride confidently to the cross pole, while having a vertical coming out gives the horse every chance to jump the fence if the horse is not quite straight. The exercise should start with the rider jumping a cross pole with a placing pole 8 ft (2.4 m) in front of it. The centre of the cross should be about 2 ft 6 in (0.7 m) high. The bounce jump wings should be

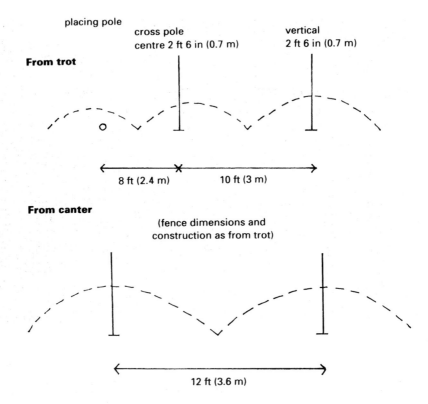

placing pole

cross pole
centre 2 ft 6 in (0.7 m)

vertical
2 ft 6 in (0.7 m)

From trot

8 ft (2.4 m)   10 ft (3 m)

From canter

(fence dimensions and
construction as from trot)

12 ft (3.6 m)

Fig. 7.13 Introducing the bounce showing distances.

in place about 10 ft (3 m) from the cross pole. The rider should be encouraged to keep the horse moving forward in trot to the placing pole so that he or she gets the feel of the horse bouncing the pole, jumping the cross pole and landing in canter. The canter should be maintained away from the fence and the horse then brought smoothly to trot. Even when jumping from trot the rider must stay in a light balanced seat, so the rider can either stay rising or stay poised with the seat lightly brushing the saddle, but the rider must *not* sit in the saddle. Ideally the exercise is set up on both sides of the school so that it can be jumped on both reins. After two or three jumps in either direction the vertical can be put up at about 2 ft 6 in (0.7 m) so that the rider has to bounce through the exercise. The rider should be able to stay in balance and keep the horse balanced on landing (Fig. 7.14).

Once the rider is confident in trot, canter can be introduced. The placing pole should be taken away and the distance between the cross pole and the vertical increased to 12 ft (3.6 m). The height and construction of the fences

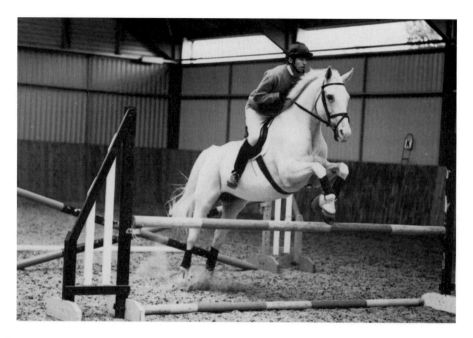

Fig. 7.14 Introducing the bounce.

should be kept the same. The rider now knows that the horse can bounce and should be confident to present the horse to the fence in its normal, rhythmic, balanced canter.

The use of Bloks or cavaletti for these exercises is not recommended because they are rather unstable and can frighten the horse if they collapse noisily in a heap. Pyramid-type jumpkins are, however, useful for grid work as they have proper plastic cups and are light and easily manoeuvrable. Using oil drums is more hazardous and best avoided.

A variety of gymnastic grids can now be used, from both trot and canter, to develop the rider's agility (Fig. 7.15).

Canter placing poles

To develop further the rider's awareness of the horse's take-off zone, cantering to a pole in front of the fence is a good exercise. For most riders it is best to keep the pole at a distance where the horse canters over the pole and then takes one non-jumping stride before the fence. The distance will vary from about 16.5 ft to 20 ft (5 to 6 m), if the pole is initially placed at 18 ft (5.5 m), the teacher can alter the distance to suit the individual horse. As the rider becomes more advanced he or she can canter to a bounce pole, but this is too much to expect the developing rider to attempt. A pole can be placed one non-jumping canter stride at the start of a grid (Fig. 7.15). If the horse does break into trot a disaster is unlikely as there is plenty of recovery time. However, if the rider has practised with ground poles sufficiently this exercise should hold few terrors.

Throughout all this work the teacher should keep a constant check on the rider, ensuring that his or her position does not lapse during this development work.

The next related distance to introduce is four strides. For training purposes the distance between the two fences is about 57–59 ft (17.3–18 m). Any combination of spread and vertical fences can be used as there is sufficient recovery time if a mistake should be made at the first fence. The main purpose is to develop further the rider's awareness of rhythm and stride control.

Once all these exercises have been completed several times to the satisfaction of both teacher and pupil, the horse and rider are probably ready to venture out to a small competition. Of course in the real world many riders

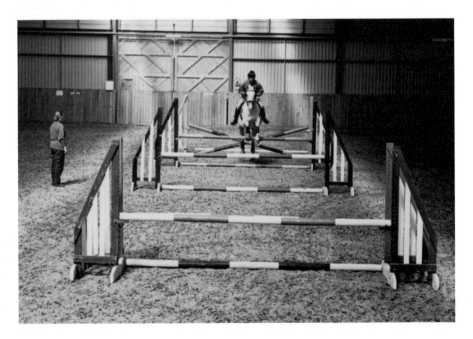

Fig. 7.15 Grid work.

go to a show never having had any instruction whatsoever. The progressive exercises outlined here show the ideal for the dedicated career rider; in many cases the teacher will have to adapt this ideal to meet the needs of individual clients.

The class lesson

The teacher may have to take a class jumping lesson , for example with pre-Stage II pupils. Here the teacher must work with distances that are correct for the majority; the distances given in Chapter 3 are usually adequate unless ponies are being used.

Most horses and riders benefit from being kept on the move most of the time. It is not recommended that the riders in a class lesson are lined up and called out to jump one at a time. This gives them little time to establish a rhythm and also allows the muscles of both horse and rider to cool down resulting in some loss of performance. There may be specific times when it is beneficial for pupils to watch and comment on each other, but sufficient warm-up time must be allowed if this technique is being used. How the riders are kept occupied while one jumps depends on the area being used and the level of the pupils. Pre-Stage II and Pony Club 'C' test riders should be capable of cantering together, but the instructor should keep the riders in walk and encourage them to pick up canter as their turn approaches, thus encouraging independent and forward thinking. Riders should *never* be allowed to jump unless the teacher is watching nor should they follow directly behind each other.

As with all teaching the position of the instructor is very important. The instructor should identify what he or she wants to see and position him or herself accordingly.

The child rider or Pony Club rider

Take for example the child with his own pony who is a Pony Club member and has instruction on a regular basis in between rallies and is taken to shows by his parents. Here the teacher's psychological and diplomatic skills will have to come into play. The teacher will have to weigh up each individual's circumstances to decide how much and where to compromise the ideal teaching plan. This compromise may be measured financially or in terms of the principles of training.

The first task is to establish the long- and short-term goals. Ideally the instructor and the child will be able to do this together and start to build up some rapport. However, the parents very often wish to be involved as well. This is quite acceptable providing that they do not dominate the discussion, in other words the instructor must try to discover what the child wants to do. Throughout, the teacher should emphasise that classical training will always enhance performance. Explain, in simple terms, why the rider who has a good position can be of more help to his or her pony and that the better trained pony can maximise its potential and last longer both physically and mentally.

In this situation it is often necessary to break the lesson down into three or four parts, for example:

(1)   Warm up on the flat
      During this time the pony and rider should be thoroughly warmed up and at the same time an aspect of the flat work can be worked on and improved. To emphasise the importance of this part it can be compared with the way the human athlete would warm up.

(2)   Warm up over small fences
      Warming up over small fences gives the instructor a chance to make some positional corrections, linking the flat work to the jumping.

(3)   Development work or problem solving
      This is the part that the child and parents will be anxious to reach, but unless parts (1) and (2) have been adequate it will be difficult to make progress. The type of work may include correcting technique or straightness or it may be that the rider wants to move up a class and feels that he or she would like some practice over larger obstacles.

(4)   Conclusion
      The lesson should finish on a positive note with feedback and evaluation from both rider and teacher. Finally the pupil should be given some 'homework' so that the pupil has a plan to work on before the next lesson.

Problems can arise when either the parents or the Pony Club team trainer have what appears to be totally opposite views. When this happens the teacher must not condemn these different views, but should try to find some positive links between the two schools of thought without shifting his or her own ground. It is important to be confident in your own system and to be positive during discussion, even if you have to go away and confirm certain points afterwards. The teacher must always remember that it is he or she who is in charge of the lesson even though the goal and the lesson plan were decided through discussion. Finish on a good moment and do not let the pupil or parent coerce you into letting them have 'one more go'. More often than not you will regret it.

The Riding Club rider

The Riding Club rider, either at home or a rally, can provide a challenge to a teacher as it is possible that the rider and/or the horse has developed undesirable habits before seeking help. It is essential to tackle these problems without undermining the confidence of the rider. It is frequently better to err on the side of caution and avoid jumping large fences. The exercises outlined earlier can be used as a positive way to solve any problems.

Riders must be encouraged to be positive in their own evaluation of their performance; use the positive to improve the negative.

An example might be that a rider has a horse that is inclined to rush. Although the rider is not frightened by this he or she knows that it can lead to the horse knocking down fences in competition. Initially the teacher can ask the rider to evaluate the problem, perhaps by giving it a mark out of ten, with one out of ten being almost impossible to ride. The rider thinks that the problem is pretty bad and gives it four out of ten. The teacher can then use some exercises to improve rushing which might include circling away from the fence and placing poles. The rider should then be asked to re-evaluate the problem; even if he or she gives it four-and-a-half out of ten there has been some improvement. Any improvement, however slight, is progress. The teacher will probably have also used the exercises as an opportunity to correct the rider's position. It is also useful to discuss the root cause of the problem – has the horse always rushed? does the horse always do it?

The horse's tack and physique should be discussed as well. Without doubt the teacher has to be prepared to be honest with the pupil, but any potentially hurtful observations must be made with tact and diplomacy. Remember that the rider may be very fond of the horse and have a somewhat different attitude to criticism of his or her horse than the competition rider. The worst situation is when the horse appears to be lame and yet the rider is totally unaware of the problem. A way to tackle this could be:

Teacher: How does your horse feel today?
Client: Fine
Teacher: May I sit on him? He looks a little uncomfortable, I might be able to feel if this is so.
Client: OK, but he doesn't feel any different to normal.

This gives the teacher the opportunity to draw the pupil's attention to what he or she is feeling when riding the horse. If the pupil can then see the lameness and agrees to discuss the problem the way forward is relatively easy. However, if the pupil cannot see or refuses to acknowledge that there is anything wrong there are two paths of action: the teacher can accept that there is nothing he or she can do about it, or if it is a serious problem the teacher may have to suggest a change of instructor. This is a matter that only the teacher and his or her conscience can decide.

The weekend rider

The weekend rider who rides perhaps once or twice a week may not have the ambition to be a top rider, but there is no reason why this rider should not be encouraged to attain the best standards possible within his or her own limitations. Even if they are not competitive these riders often like to have their achievements recognised, thus 'in-house competence tests' are often well received. In other words, the teacher can set up an exercise that allows the riders to demonstrate their competence; each test can be tailormade to suit the individual rider.

Record cards

It is strongly recommended that teachers keep record cards which chart the riders' progress, which horses they have ridden, which instructors were involved and the goals set and achieved. Clients can be invited to keep these cards up-to-date, so becoming involved in their own learning as well as relieving the teacher of some of the paperwork. Many gyms and fitness centres operate this sort of system so that if a trainer has to cover for someone else's clients he or she knows what is happening.

Summary

- Overall aim: to develop the rider's ability to maintain the quality of the work at all times.
- By developing:
  self-awareness
  discipline
  feel for the horse
  confidence
  increasing knowledge.
- Method
  developing rhythm and balance on the flat
  introducing rhythmic cantering over ground poles and fences
  developing athleticism through grids and gymnastic exercises
  introducing the concept of riding a line through a course of fences.
- The tools of the trade
  the horse – how to choose the horse – matching horse and rider
  equipment – types of jump – how to use them efficiently.
- Transferring skills
  when and how to compromise
  the child rider or Pony Club rider
  the Riding Club rider
  the weekend rider.
- Likely problems
  rider losing balance
  horse losing balance and rhythm
  lack of rider self-discipline
  rider impatience regarding progress.

8 Cross-country Training

The aim of this chapter is to introduce the concept of riding in open spaces and developing rider awareness of how natural conditions can affect the way horse and rider react. If a rider has been fortunate enough to have been brought up with horses he or she will have spent much of the time riding outdoors, but today many riders have their first experiences with horses in a riding school. Some will have had very little contact with the countryside and while everything is new and frightening to a degree the experience will also be very enriching.

There was a time when holiday-makers climbed onto quiet horses and ponies and without any more ado were taken into the countryside. Certainly the riders were able to enjoy the views, but lack of basic riding skills and an understanding of the way horses react must have taken the edge off this enjoyment due to physical discomfort and some uncertainty of their ability to control the animal on which they were mounted. These days most holiday centres do give rudimentary guidance to their clients and are encouraged to assess riders' capabilities before sending them out on a horse, whether it be for one hour or one day.

Professional instructors should seek to ensure that clients are at least able to walk, trot and canter safely in an enclosed area before letting them ride on roads, tracks or fields. Furthermore the serious rider should be developed to at least the level outlined in Chapter 7.

Introducing cross-country riding

Assuming that the rider is inexperienced, an excellent introduction to cross-country riding is to hack out in groups accompanied by a qualified instructor. Everyone who rides will have had experience with roads and traffic. If they are drivers they will have been encouraged to observe likely hazards and react accordingly. Even as a pedestrian you have to 'look before you cross' and watch out for other pedestrians and road users. All these skills are equally relevant on horseback and an ability to observe and to be alert is essential to riders and instructors. For instance, a group of riders working in the same arena have to be vigilant and aware of each other, giving way courteously and calling attention where necessary. Working-in at a competition, often in cramped conditions, requires fine tuning of these skills if an accident is to be avoided. Hacking out in groups teaches the rider first and foremost to be alert; even well-behaved horses can be startled by a plastic bag in the hedge or a pheasant flying out from under their feet. Riders must take in everything around them and try to anticipate potential problems. The instructor is there to fulfil several functions:

- to warn of possible hazards and to advise the rider how to overcome problems that he or she may be experiencing with the horse, for example turning the horse's head away from frightening objects;
- to give positional corrections that are key to improving performance, shortening the reins for example;
- to determine the speed that horse and rider tackle certain terrain and explain why that speed has been chosen;
- to explain the effects of the 'going' or the terrain on the horse – uphill, downhill, slippery, rough and hard;
- to explain the procedure for crossing fords or streams;
- to deal with traffic and explain to the riders that not all motorists are aware how quickly horses can move;
- to outline accident procedure (see Appendix 3);
- to explain the Country Code and define acceptable rider behaviour in the countryside;
- to explain how horses may react to the weather, to being ridden in company, and the signals of a less than confident rider;
- finally, and most importantly, the instructor will emphasise the need to plan ahead, especially when stopping, turning or speeding up.

In this way a simple hack in the countryside can, with a competent escort, be a very productive exercise in terms of widening the riders' experience and preparing them for jumping cross-country fences. When riding outdoors in this way it is recommended that the riders have their stirrups at jumping length, so that they can maintain a light seat when cantering across a field, for example.

Once riders have attained the level of competence outlined in Chapter 7 in an enclosed school or manege, they can progress to working in a small field or jumping paddock, about 1 ha is ideal. The trot and canter work should be with a light seat. When they are confident, other riders can join them so that they can start to experience the sensation of riding in company outside. For these early sessions it is useful if the instructor is mounted so that they can react swiftly to a situation and solve a problem before it gets out of control.

If the rider is a little nervous or the horse likely to be frisky, it is recommended that a neck strap is used to give the rider a feeling of security. The correct matching of horse and rider is very important for these early adventures outside; being out of control or feeling out of control is very frightening, even for experienced riders. Ideally the pupil should ride a horse that he or she is already familiar with. Just as in the more formal teaching environment, the rider should be encouraged to give feedback to the teacher and the teacher must constantly check that the rider is confident and happy to move on to the next stage. The rider may need reassurance from time to time and the nervous rider must not be bullied or ridiculed.

What factors make riding outside different?

The 'going'

Unlike an arena, the conditions underfoot when riding outside will vary depending on many factors including the weather, soil type, and how much use the field or track gets. Riders should be aware of this and know how the horse may react and how they can best assist the horse and hence themselves. For example, recent rain, ice, snow or very hard ground can make the surface slippery. When horses slip they tend to frighten themselves and become tense and tight in the back, so by avoiding sharp turns and 'heavy braking' the rider can help to avoid accidents and also give the horse confidence. The instructor therefore should advise the riders to slow down for turns and give plenty of warning before pulling up. In some ways a horse is like a car; if slowing down is left too late and the brakes are applied too sharply the horse may skid into the horse in front, which in turn could lead to horse or rider getting kicked.

Very wet or boggy ground has a different effect; the horse may struggle to pull its feet out of the mud and, as a consequence, stumble. The rider should be encouraged to sit as lightly as possible and let the horse take its time to pick its way through the deep patch. Rough going over rutted tracks or plough needs special care as the horse is likely to stumble or veer onto better ground. Novice riders should not be asked to canter over this sort of ground as it is difficult to stay in balance and thus easy to tumble off should the horse suddenly lurch or trip.

Gradients

The next phase for the novice rider is to experience going up- and downhill. It is better to start with going uphill in walk, trot and, finally, canter. The aim is to encourage the rider to stay in balance, neither falling onto the horse's back nor collapsing onto the neck. The neck strap can be used until the rider has developed better balance. The rider should be aware what hard work it is for the horse and how much hock engagement the horse needs to propel itself uphill. Probably the hardest thing for the rider to do is to trot uphill and remain in a balanced, light seat, but once this is mastered cantering is relatively easy (Figs 8.1 and 8.2).

Going downhill is potentially much more frightening for riders. They should be encouraged to keep the shoulders up and still maintain a light seat, not sit down in the saddle (Figs 8.3 and 8.4). However, the rider must not get too far in front of the movement or the horse will be pushed onto its

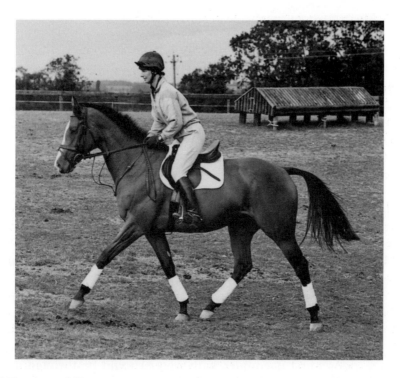

Fig. 8.1 Trotting uphill.

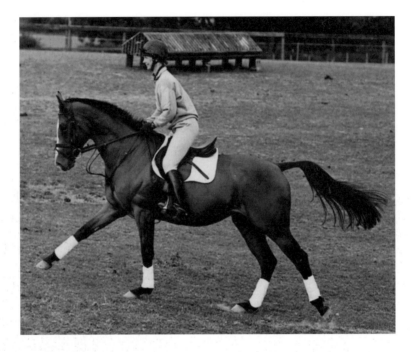

Fig. 8.2 Cantering uphill.

forehand and lose its balance. In order to do this the lower leg must be stable enough to keep the rider secure which takes some practice. Obviously it is sensible to teach the rider to ride downhill in all three paces before asking them to jump downhill.

Ridge and furrow
In some parts of the country it is common to find ridge and furrow fields. Crossing this terrain means that the horse is constantly having to adjust its balance as it goes up and down these rolling hillocks. The rider should be taught to sit as still as possible with a consistent feel down the rein. The rider should be aware that when the horse is cantering across ridge and furrow it may frequently change leading legs; the rider's job is to sit still, with the weight over the lower leg and down into the heel, and interfere as little as possible.

Water
Ideally the rider's first encounter with water should be through a ford or stream, or possibly paddling in the sea. The rider should be asked to analyse

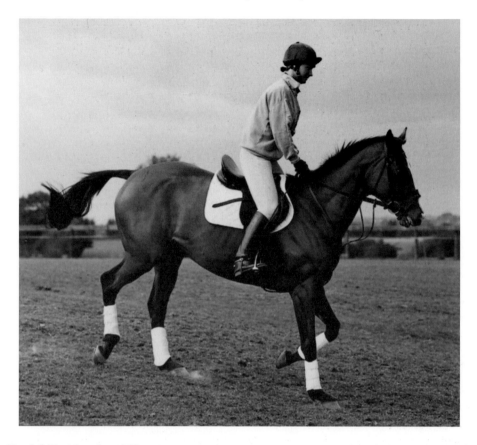

Fig. 8.3 Trotting downhill.

how he or she feels when walking in water to make him or her realise that the horse experiences the same dragging sensation and that it is hard work for the horse to work in water. The rider should also realise that the deeper the water and the faster the horse goes the more of a bow wave it creates; this can cause a problem later on if the horse is asked to jump in and out of water. If the circumstances allow, the rider can experiment by first walking the horse and then building up to cantering through the water. It is the teacher's responsibility to ensure that the bottom of the water is safe for the horse to work in and if a water crossing has not been used for some time it should be checked before using it. If the horses are being paddled in the water riders should be reminded that if a horse starts to paw at the water there is a chance that it may get down and roll so they must keep their wits about them.

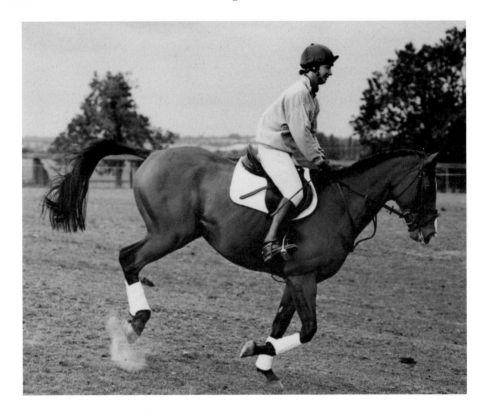

Fig. 8.4 Cantering downhill.

The horse's instincts

Normally riding outside will be taught to a group of two or more riders and group riding skills must be taught early. The pupil should be reminded that the horse is a creature of instinct and that when frightened the horse's instinct is to flee. If the rider contains that desire to run away then instead the horse may buck, rear, go sideways and otherwise evade the rider's aids. With schooling most horses learn to trust their rider so that the horse obeys the rider's aids even when frightened and being restrained. However, this is one reason why novice riders and novice horses do not make an ideal mix. The unpredictable nature of the horse also makes it essential that novice riders are accompanied when out on a hack so that the instructor can give speedy advice to minimise the trauma of a horse misbehaving.

The rider must also be aware of the horse's herd instinct. By nature horses are gregarious animals; in the wild they congregate in groups which follow a herd leader. The horse that is by nature the herd leader is often the sort that, with correct training, makes the top class hunter or event horse. The critical factor for novice riders to realise is that their horse may be reluctant to turn away and leave the others, and firm direction from the rider may be needed. However, it is crucial that riders are able to take the horse where they want, when they want; for example, when jumping the horse has to be willing to leave the others and perform on its own. If the horse is 'napping' back to the rest of the ride it will not be committed to jumping the fence, it may make an awkward jump and thus lose its confidence and that of its rider.

Another hazard that riders must be aware of when riding in groups is that horses may kick if they feel threatened by, for example, a horse passing too close behind them. This tendency is exacerbated if the horse is excited or unfamiliar with the group or if it is a mare in season. All riders must know that the usual one-and-a-half horses' length distance that is kept when riding in the manege should be doubled when riding outside. If riding side by side riders must watch out for the horses showing signs of distrust, such as the ears going back. Vulnerable moments occur when queueing to go through gateways or following down narrow tracks. Horses can also become excited when turning for home at the end of a session, taking advantage of their rider being relaxed and less vigilant.

Evaluating performance

The instructor should spend several sessions working the riders in groups yet with each rider having an individual project. This exercise should start in trot and then progress to canter when the riders are sufficiently confident and capable. This method also allows each rider to progress at a speed that is best for him or her. The instructor has to be very vigilant and ready to change a rider onto a different horse if the rider is experiencing difficulty. One of the problems facing the instructor is being heard and although audio aids are improving they are still expensive and not all types can be used when mounted.

Once the riders have carried out their assigned tasks the instructor should ask the pupils to evaluate how their horses have performed.

- Did the horse settle well?
- Was it keen or lazy?
- Did it feel even on both reins?

- Did it lead on the appropriate leg or did it become unbalanced and change legs or become disunited?
- How fit did the horse seem?
- Did it blow excessively on pulling up?
- Were there any signs of lameness or discomfort?
- Did the horse hang back from the other horses or towards home?

The riders should also do some self-evaluation.

- Did they enjoy the work?
- Were they always in control?
- Were there times when they became unbalanced?
- Did they ache or become breathless?
- What would they like to do next?

Galloping

Once the rider has become secure and confident galloping can be introduced. The gallop is the horse's fastest and most extended pace. The diagonal sequence of the canter is broken so that all four hoof beats can be heard followed by a moment of suspension. The sequence of footfalls for gallop with left fore lead is:

right hind – left hind – right fore – left fore.

As with canter it is important that the following are maintained in gallop:

- rhythm
- even, unhurried strides
- straightness.

To a novice rider the gallop will feel very fast and should be introduced by gradually increasing the speed of the canter until the horse is galloping without the rider really being aware that anything significant has happened. However, as the average horse is unlikely to be galloping until it reaches a speed of about 20 miles per hour (580–600 m per minute) much room will be needed to teach the rider to gallop. Sharp turns and steep slopes must be avoided. It may be useful for the serious rider to hire the use of an all-weather gallop from a racehorse trainer. Galloping is best taught on a one-to-one basis so that the teacher can be mounted and ride 'upsides' with the pupil, talking the pupil through the exercise. If the pupil has thoroughly mastered cantering in balance then the progression to galloping is relatively easy, but the pupil does need plenty of practice and help before embarking on any form of competitive galloping.

The pupil should shorten the stirrups to a length where he or she can stay in balance and yet still be able to use his or her legs effectively. The difference in length between flat work and jumping will vary according to the rider's experience, length of leg and type of saddle, for example the event rider Blyth Tait would ride five or six holes shorter for galloping. The teacher should explain to the pupils why they have to shorten their stirrups and they will be able to find out for themselves that the horse's centre of gravity moves further forward as the speed increases. Initially the novice rider will feel quite insecure with short stirrups, but it is all a matter of practice; youngsters who attend the British Racing School at Newmarket learn to gallop a racehorse in eight weeks, many never having ridden before. Their stirrups are fairly short at the outset and by the time the course finishes are very short indeed, by normal standards. The key point for the pupil to grasp is that the rider's weight must never bump in the saddle and the lower leg must remain stable with a lowered heel. The rider who is just learning to gallop is probably happiest holding the reins in the normal way but short enough to be able to react quickly if necessary. Later the rider can be taught to 'bridge' the reins, which is especially helpful with a strong pulling horse.

Rider fitness

Before riders consider competing in any cross-country event, even a hunter trial, they should be able to gallop for at least a mile without getting tired. Pupils should be asked to gauge their fitness in terms of legache, backache or breathlessness. One of the benefits of riding, even for the leisure rider, is that it promotes a degree of physical fitness. Riding is aerobic exercise that strengthens the rider's heart and lungs and helps to burn body fat, particularly if the riding is prolonged or at speed. It teaches the rider to breathe properly – how often does the teacher say to the pupil, 'Don't forget to breathe'? Added to this, spending time in the fresh air is therapeutic in itself.

Riders need to become fit so that they can be of maximum help to their horses, not a hindrance. The activity of riding tones up the bottom, legs and inner thighs as well as strengthening the stomach and lower back muscles. If in addition the rider can be persuaded to work-out at a gym, swim or cycle the extra fitness will help their riding skills.

Cross-country gear

The pupil must have the correct attire for riding cross-country. The hat should be of the latest BSI or European Standard. Safe boots should have a clearly defined heel and smooth sole. Body protectors give additional safety and if the pupil wishes to compete in affiliated Horse Trials or take BHS examinations a body protector is mandatory. There is a great range to choose from and the correct choice will depend on the rider's personal taste as well as his or her riding ambitions. Most riders find that gloves are essential, for warmth in cold weather and to help grip the reins when the horse becomes hot and sweaty.

Warming up and cooling down

The instructor must ensure that riders are aware of the importance of warming the horse up correctly, with at least 20 minutes of walking and trotting before the horse is asked to canter or gallop. Once the work is finished the rider should be taught to pull the horse up gradually so that it stays in balance. Sudden changes of pace can be very stressful to the tendons and ligaments of the lower leg. The horse must then be thoroughly cooled down before returning to the stable; depending on the amount of work done, this is likely to take about 20 minutes. The instructor must remember to build adequate warming up and cooling down time into the lesson plan.

The concept that the rider is aware of the horse's physical needs adds an extra dimension of enjoyment to the whole riding experience, whatever the rider's aims. The rider may simply be riding occasionally for pleasure or may intend to make riding a career; either way the instructor should constantly seek to educate his or her charge.

The voice

Any teacher, be it in a classroom or a field, needs to take care of his or her voice, as once damaged it may never fully recover. A person's voice is affected by physical build and habits of speech which are determined by childhood influences. On the whole the individuality of speech is attractive, but the instructor must take care not to let his or her voice become too high in an attempt to be heard as a shriek does not have an effective carrying capacity. On the other hand if the voice tends to drop towards the end of a sentence valuable words may be lost to the pupil. The riding instructor needs to train the voice to give greater range, flexibility and carrying power. There are a few basic guidelines to follow which will help:

- Stand with the weight evenly distributed on the ball of the foot and the heel.
- If sitting do not strain forwards as the alignment of the breathing apparatus is not at its most effective in this position.
- In the same way that the pupil is reminded to breathe evenly and deeply, so should the teacher.
- Take time to say the key words, especially in the open.
- If the rider is a long way away a stream of comments, commands and corrections will not be heard; keep any words simple.
- Reserve longer discussions for times when the rider is closer.
- Each individual should try to find his or her own pitch level which makes the most efficient use of the voice. To find the natural pitch of the voice, say 'hmhm' as if in agreement; this can then be enhanced.
- Face the person that is being addressed. Teaching on the outside of a circle or square makes this easier.
- Keep the voice lubricated (not with alcohol!) as a dry throat can quickly lead to strain.
- If suffering from a cough or cold, keep talking to a minimum, as this is when the voice will be most susceptible to long-term damage. Try to avoid clearing the throat; it is better to take a sip of water and swallow it silently. Sucking fruit pastilles can also keep the mouth moist and make voice production easier.
- Practise how much the voice can be lowered and still carry.
- Practise putting expression into the voice to convey enthusiasm, concern, encouragement and reprimand. Remember, sound can only come out effectively if the mouth is open!

The shy teacher can practise training the voice in the bath or the car. He or she will soon find out if, for example, the voice becomes too high and this can then be corrected. There are experts in the field of voice production and care; those with problems should refer to them. Remember, the teacher's voice is the most important tool of the trade and it should be taken care of.

Summary

- Overall aim: to introduce the pupil to riding in the countryside.
- By:
    having a structured plan which is carried out step by step
    using a small paddock of about 1 ha
    hacking out on tracks, trails and bridle paths
    using cross-country training areas and hills
    encouraging independent riding
    galloping.
- Method
    Educating the rider in:
    - horse psychology
    - countryside lore
    - effect of weather
    - terrain, going and location
    - rules of riding in company
    - accident procedures
    Practising riding at all three paces uphill, downhill, through water and over varying terrain and going:
    - coping with wayward horses
    - group riding skills, coping with varying abilities and needs
    - awareness of horse fitness and welfare.
- The tools of the trade
    environment – choosing a venue
    the voice – as an artificial aid, care and production.
- Likely problems
    fear of riding in the open; the rider does not feel in control
    does the rider trust the horse?
    does the rider have confidence in the trainer?

9 Introducing the Rider to Cross-country Jumps

The aim of this chapter is to outline how to introduce the rider to jumping cross-country fences. The earlier training should have resulted in a secure, balanced rider who is keen to progress to cross-country. As cross-country courses have become more technical horses are asked to be more accurate; this means that the rider also has to be able to ride more accurately. Practice over narrow fences is invaluable with emphasis being placed on straightness and rhythm with a positive forward thinking approach that does not involve extra speed. Three of the most important aspects of cross-country riding are:

- to develop the ability to keep the horse consistently in balance;
- to be able to jump the fence accurately;
- to know the optimum speed and to be able to regulate it.

Even though at this early stage the measurement of speed is not a concern, the underlying principles of cross-country riding remain the same.

The vital ingredients

From the outset it must be stressed that the horse must be safe, honest and controllable. Furthermore the rider must feel confident about the horse; this confidence will stem from the rider's previous experience with that horse as well as the size and behaviour of the horse being such that the rider feels secure. The other vital component is that the rider has already had lessons with the instructor and that they have built up a rapport. The instructor should know the pupil well enough to ascertain whether he or she is afraid, nervous or simply unsure. For early cross-country experience it is ideal to work with a group of riders; riders generally feel more confident if there are others 'having a go'.

Should the instructor be mounted?

Whether or not the instructor should be mounted is a matter of personal taste and can depend on a variety of factors, for example the venue may involve a hack or a journey in a horsebox. By this time, having followed the training programme, the instructor should be confident that the pupils are confident of hacking to the venue without direct supervision.

The advantages of the instructor being mounted include the ability to:

- talk to the riders throughout;
- get to the scene of a problem quickly;
- demonstrate how to ride a particular fence.

The disadvantages of the instructor being mounted arise:

- if the instructor has to check a fence on foot; somebody will be needed to hold the horse;
- if the instructor has to get on a pupil's horse to correct it or demonstrate to the rider;
- in the event of an accident it is one more horse to cope with and in all probability there will only be pupils present, no helpers on foot;
- if the instructor's horse is a school horse, it means that horse is not earning money.

As a compromise, or perhaps an ideal, there should be another rider in the group who is experienced enough to act as an escort and a demonstrator.

Choice of venue

As has been emphasised throughout, quality of work is the aim and the measurable objective is the achievement of that quality. It will not be possible to achieve the objective unless the facilities are suitable. The choice of venue will depend on the experience and expertise of the riders. For the introduction to cross-country fences it is ideal to have a group of fences in a small area, perhaps 1 ha. The fences should not exceed 2 ft 9 in (0.8 m), making them small enough for both horses and ponies. It is very important that the going is safe; if there is any doubt about the suitability of the going the riders should initially ride in the area without jumping. If the horses are slipping and sliding and losing confidence then the going is not suitable for introducing novice riders to this new venture. The fences should be well constructed and solid and inviting. Ideally the take-off and landing should be an all-weather surface or well maintained; rutted and poached ground can result in the horse stumbling on take-off or landing and there being an accident to horse or rider.

The instructor has the total responsibility for ensuring that the fences are safe and suitable. Never school over cross-country fences if there are loose horses in the field; indeed teaching should never take place in such circumstances.

Warm up

Allow at least 15–20 minutes warm up in trot and canter, during which time the instructor can check the position and balance of the riders. The riders must be alert as to the whereabouts of each other and act responsibly. Once the horses and riders are warmed up the instructor can ask for some feedback.

- How has the warm up gone?
- Can the riders control their horses?
- Is the tack safe and suitable?
- Are the riders confident?

The lesson plan

The instructor should then explain the plan for the lesson. Thirty minutes of actual jump training is likely to be sufficient, so the lesson format will be:

- Warm up for 15–20 minutes to include mounting and hacking to the venue.
- Jump training for 30 minutes.
- Cool down for 10–15 minutes.

As with all training the riders should be kept on the move most of the time. It is important that the horse's muscles do not cool down and become stiff otherwise problems may occur when the horse is asked to do something strenuous.

The first two fences

The riders should start over a simple first fence (Fig. 9.1). A log is ideal; however, tyres are also suitable, providing that the horse is used to them. As most riders have an innate fear of losing control it is a good idea to start by approaching the fence in trot. The rider can be encouraged to land in canter, stay in balance, make a smooth transition to trot and then jump the log again. Once the rider is confident, the horse can be asked to stay in canter on landing and come round to the fence in canter. The canter should be the rhythmic balanced canter that has been practised in all the previous jump training. Once the riders have jumped the fence from canter a couple of times they can be stopped and asked to evaluate the work so far. The

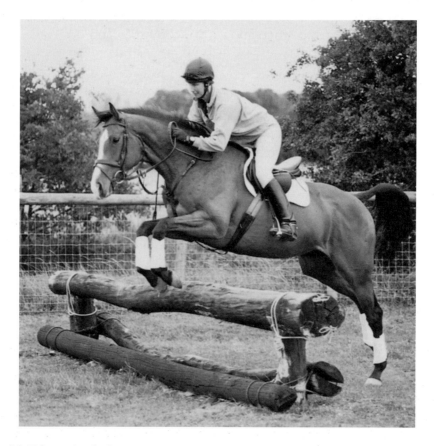

Fig. 9.1 Using a simple fence to start.

instructor can then correct them as necessary and move on to the next exercise.

The next fence should also be an easy one such as a post and rails, small gate, sleepers or a pheasant feeder. As their turn to jump approaches the riders should be encouraged to pick up canter, check that the canter is of good quality, count the rhythm, pop the fence, land in balance, canter away, turn and come to the fence again. At this stage only one horse should be allowed to jump at one time and only when the instructor has a clear view.

The rider's lower leg

At this stage the riders will probably feel most comfortable with their stirrups at their usual jumping length. The instructor must be most diligent regarding the rider's lower leg; any tendency for it to slip back will lead to instability. As the riders progress to the next easy fence they can be asked to concentrate on their lower leg: is it effective? is it stable?

Control

The horses often begin to get a little keen and the instructor may need to give the riders some advice on how to restrain them. Check that the rider is not getting overexcited and encouraging the horse to become overkeen. The rider's reins must be short enough and there should not be excessive hand and body movement over the fence. The instructor should explain to the riders that the horse can be circled to slow it down, but not at the expense of it losing its balance or footing. If the rider has serious doubts about his or her ability to control the horse then the rider should be changed onto a different horse or drop out of the lesson. Experience shows that once a rider feels out of control it is only a matter of time before he or she really is out of control and that is frightening for all concerned.

Ditches

The riders should now be ready to jump a small ditch. The ditch should be a simple, small open ditch, no more than 3ft (1m) wide. From the outset it is important that the rider realises that all ditches have to be ridden firmly but in rhythm and that the horse must be kept straight. It should be explained that horses often slow down, possibly 'spooking', before jumping a ditch. Even though these fences are small the riders should be encouraged to look up, especially where ditches and drops are concerned. If a plain open ditch is not available a tiger trap or trakhener would be a suitable second choice. This type of fence encourages the rider to approach in a stronger rhythm, which is a good goal to be striving for, but the word 'rhythm' must be accentuated. Riding more strongly to a fence does not mean just going faster.

The finish

Finish each cross-country session on a good note; do not leave the most difficult fence until last. The instructor's plan will have to be flexible and he or she must monitor the progress of each rider to ensure the best long-term benefit.

Subsequent lessons

If the next lesson is at the same venue, having warmed up, the riders could jump two or three easy fences from the last lesson as a jumping warm up. They may do this in open order in which case the instructor must ensure that the riders know which fences are being jumped and from which direction, to avoid the risk of collisions.

The riders can progress to jumping combinations, which may be as simple as a post and rails double or as complex as a coffin. Ideally the lesson would start with a post and rails double. The instructor should check the riders' lower leg positions and their maintenance of balance. If the riders are asked to imagine that the first rail is part of a coffin this will help ensure that the horse is in front of the leg and that the rhythm and take-off point is consistent.

Coffins

However simple the construction of the coffin, riders must be taught the correct principles for jumping it from the outset. The instructor should explain the effect of the ditch on the horse and consequently on the rider. Take care that the rider does not get in front of the movement, and although a light contact with the mouth is ideal, it should never be a backward pull.

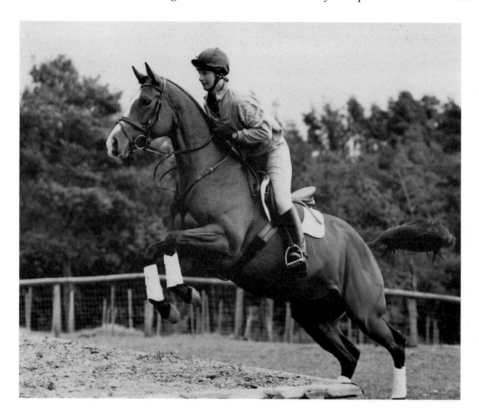

Fig. 9.2 Jumping up a bank.

Banks

When the rider is being taught to jump banks the instructor should stress the need to have the horse thinking forwards (Fig. 9.2). Ideally the bank will allow the horse to take a stride on top to give the rider a chance to recover his or her position. However, if it is simply a bounce the rider must try to stay as still as possible with the lower leg close to the horse's sides and not sliding back. As the horse jumps off the bank the rider should keep the shoulders up and then allow the horse as much head and neck room as is wanted, keeping the weight balanced over the lower leg (Fig. 9.3). Often at this stage the rider bumps into the saddle; if this happens the rider should be encouraged to regain a balanced seat as soon as possible without disturbing the horse's balance.

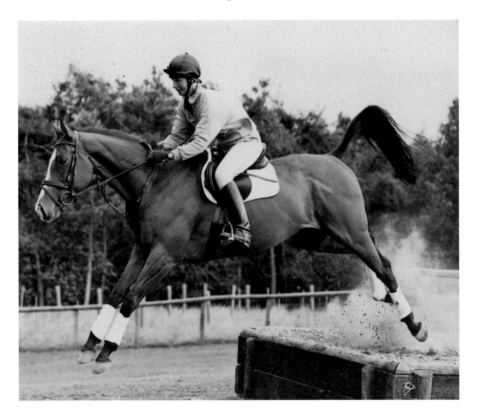

Fig. 9.3 Jumping off a bank, keeping the lower leg secure and allowing with the rein.

Steps

Once the rider is confident over a bank and can stay in balance with relative ease, steps, both up and down, can be introduced. The approach to steps up should be a strong, rhythmic but controlled canter. As the horse jumps up the rider should go forward with the horse, maintaining the rein contact and keeping the horse straight at each element. As the horse reaches the top it will need to be gathered together and put back into the balanced canter to approach the next obstacle.

Going down steps the rider needs to steady the horse a little, keeping the legs on and maintaining a light elastic contact. As the horse descends each step the rider's shoulders should be kept back a little and the weight kept over the lower leg so that the horse can drop down as smoothly as possible, land and get away in balance (Fig. 9.4). Often these downhill fences encour-

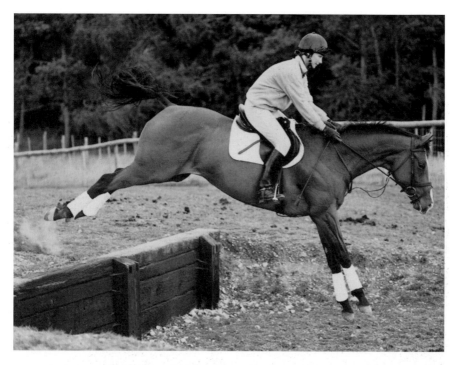

Fig. 9.4 Allowing with the hand while keeping the body weight over the centre of balance.

age the rider to flop forwards, putting extra weight onto the horse's forehand so that the horse rushes away at the bottom.

The getaway

The instructor must emphasise the importance of both the getaway from the fence and the balance in-between the fences. At more advanced levels where time and speed are vital to success, an efficient getaway from a fence will save valuable seconds without having to rush or fluster the horse.

Water

By now the pupil should be ready to tackle water. If the training programme has been followed then the pupil should have ridden through streams out hacking (Figs 9.5 and 9.6), but it is a good idea to do some revision and

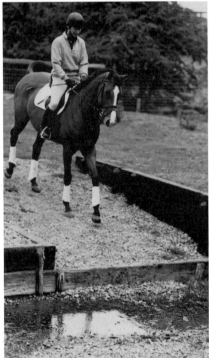

9.5

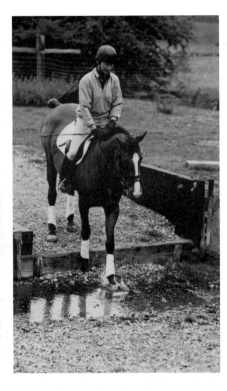

9.6

Figs 9.5 and 9.6 Introducing water.

ask the rider what to do when jumping down a small step into water and riding away out of the water up a slope. The answers should include:

- keep the horse sufficiently forward from the leg to the hand;
- maintain the rein contact;
- realise that the water will 'drag' the horse;
- not rush the horse through the water;
- keep the horse together in the best possible balance.

Once the step down into water has been mastered, the exercise can be Swapped around so that the horse enters the water down the slope and leaves by jumping out of the water up the step (Fig. 9.7). The same principles apply to jumping a step out of water as jumping up steps on dry land, but the rider must be warned that the horse can trip up the step if it misses its footing in the water or slips on landing. By now the rider's position should be quite secure and if this happens he or she should only be temporarily unbalanced. Horses hate their riders falling off; it makes them lose confidence which is one of the reasons why this 'step by step' approach is recommended.

Once the rider is confident with this exercise then a step down into water followed by a step out of the water can be introduced. The next stage would be to introduce a jump two or three strides away from the water to be jumped either on the approach to the water or the exit from the water.

The riders should be encouraged to think for themselves. They can be asked, for example, how they think their horse might react to jumping a log followed two strides later by water. If the riders have learned from their experiences of jumping coffin-type fences they should realise that the horse is likely to 'back off' and will need reassurance from the rider. The rider

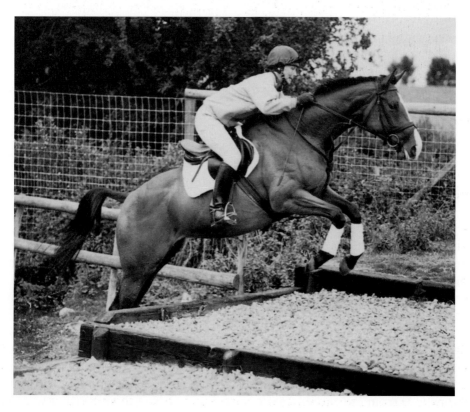

Fig. 9.7 Step up out of water.

should also realise the possible dangers of landing unbalanced at a fence before water. Essentially once the rider loses balance the horse is in control; the honest schoolmaster horse will probably help the rider out, but the instructor must be quick to spot if this is the case and repeat the exercise until sufficient improvement has been made.

In the same way, the instructor can ask the riders what they would do if their horse made a mistake coming up a step out of water with a post and rails two strides away. The rider's answer should depend on the severity of the mistake. If during a training session the horse had tripped and fallen onto its knees it would probably be wise to pull the horse out from the fence. If the horse had simply lost impulsion and landed up the step in a heap the rider should use his or her legs vigorously to initiate some impulsion. Jumping out of water and then a related fence is not easy; the rider will have to practise being able to 'stay with' the horse and it is easy to get behind the movement. For this reason it is essential that these early training fences are small, well built and not narrow or 'trappy'. The novice cross-country rider is not yet able to influence the horse sufficiently to be able to jump arrowheads or similar fences in a complicated situation. Fences requiring accuracy should be introduced separately on flat ground and the technique further refined by school exercises as described in Chapter 16.

When teaching the rider to jump a fence actually in the water he or she should be encouraged to ride the horse firmly but not fast to the obstacle. The rider should be ready to recover quickly if the horse makes a mistake by keeping the shoulders up and the lower leg secure.

Slopes

By the third training session the rider may be ready to tackle fences situated either before or after a slope, for example a post and rails placed 21 ft (6.4 m) before going down a steep slope. Again at the beginning of the session the pupils can be asked what they think is going to happen and how they feel this fence should be tackled. If the slope is into a dark wooded area the pupils should be expected to realise that this will affect the situation; the horse may be hesitant to go into the dark unknown territory and may need extra back-up from the rider's leg as they approach the rails; however, the horse must not become fast or unbalanced. The riders must also be aware that going down the slope will put the horse onto the forehand and should use the knowledge from the earlier training sessions to adjust their position to cope with the problem. If the rail is at the bottom of the slope the problem is one of balance. Provided that the rider keeps the horse balanced down the slope and does not 'hustle' the horse to the fence but 'waits' for the take-off all will be well. If, however, the rider becomes too far behind the horse's movement coming down the slope and the horse rushes to the rail the rider is likely to be badly 'left behind' and both horse and rider will have an uncomfortable experience.

At this stage both pupil and teacher will begin to realise the value of teaching the rider how to cope with the terrain before beginning to jump cross-country fences.

Fences on a downhill slope are probably the most awesome for the novice rider so it is essential that they are small and easy to jump, for example a log or sloping palisade is much more inviting than an upright. The rider must be encouraged to keep the lower leg at or slightly in front of the girth, the shoulders and upper body should be more or less upright and the reins slipped as much as the horse requires. Provided that the rider has not become too unbalanced, retrieving the reins and rebalancing is just a matter of practice and becomes almost automatic with time. To become adept at this manoeuvre it is essential not to proceed to more difficult fences or steeper slopes until the rider is confident. The technique for landing over a drop fence is only a variation on this; however, if the drop fence is combined with a further problem more care has to be taken on the approach. A drop fence is complicated by:

- jumping from light into dark, for example fence three at Gatcombe Park, Gloucestershire is a wall into a wood, landing on a steep slope with upright rails at the bottom, a very difficult jump;
- landing in water – the water drags the horse's legs making landing more hazardous;
- a bank with a jump off (Normandy Bank). The jump off may be a log at novice level or rails at advanced level; either way the rider must be aware that there will be jarring and a loss of momentum on landing and thus of the need for maintaining a secure position.

Another type of drop fence is the sunken road which is a variation on a coffin. The ideal introduction to this sort of fence is a simple drop down off a bank or down a step which gives the horse time to balance itself, make the bounce or one stride as required and then jump up the next bank or step. In this simple form, the rider uses the technique already outlined for the drop down but on landing has to quickly get the body forward, pick up a light rein contact and close the legs to maintain the forward momentum. This enables the rider to stay in the most effective position throughout. Of course the rider's position will not always be perfect; especially if the horse does anything unusual the rider is likely to get left behind jumping up the step. The most important thing is to remind the rider not to pull on the reins and to 'get his or her act together' as quickly as possible after the incident. This would be particularly important if there was another jump close to the jump out of the sunken road. Once the rider is competent and confident jumping through a simple sunken road he or she can progress to a combination where there is a fence before the step down which may be sited so that the horse either lands and bounces down the drop or takes one stride. In both cases the rider needs to be quite well advanced before he or she could be expected to stay in balance throughout.

There are many types of drop fence and as the rider's experience grows he or she will recognise the problems that each poses and be able to react accordingly.

Uphill fences

Uphill fences are relatively easy, requiring lots of energy; they are jumped in a similar way to going up steps or a bank. Horses rarely make mistakes at uphill fences unless they are seriously short of power so the instructor needs to make the pupil aware of keeping a strong rhythmic canter with the seat out of the saddle and the rein contact maintained. Sometimes the rider may experience difficulty in staying in balance if the horse takes off earlier than anticipated.

Accuracy fences

Increasingly cross-country courses include fences that require accurate riding of a line on approach. Ideally the rider is introduced to small corners and arrowheads while cross-country schooling. If this is not possible the instructor can build similar fences in the manege as described in Chapter 16.

Corners (Fig. 9.8)

The first corner that a rider is asked to jump should have a substantial wing such as a tree or a bush; it should also have a bush planted at a spot that will

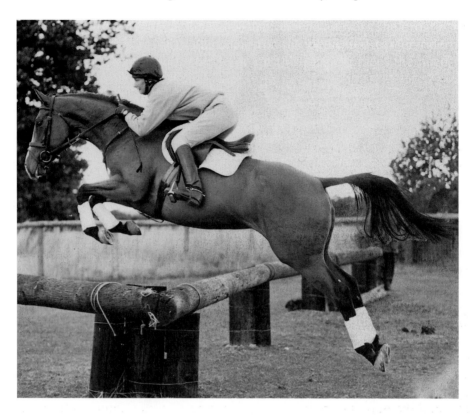

Fig. 9.8 Corner.

deter the horse from jumping part of the corner that is too wide. The rider should understand the principle of jumping a corner. Ideally the horse should jump across a corner at 90° to an imaginary line that bisects the angle of the corner (Fig. 9.9). Having decided which part of the fence to jump, the rider should find a landmark behind the fence to look for on the approach to the fence. The rider should then go to the landing side of the fence, turn his or her back on the landmark and determine whether the chosen line matches up. It is vital for the novice rider to be able to pick up a suitable line six or seven strides (59–69 ft 18–21 m) away from the fence. If possible it is helpful to paint a spot on the fence marking where you want the rider to aim for. This will encourage the rider to develop accuracy by giving him or her confidence of which part of the fence to tackle.

Once the line is determined the rider must make sure that he or she has the right quality of canter – strong, contained and rhythmic. The teacher

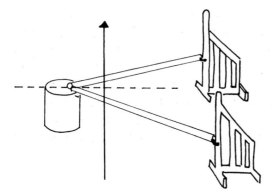

Fig. 9.9 How to jump a corner.

must not forget to encourage the riders to tell the teacher what they feel they need. Riders should be corrected as necessary and the teacher must always be prepared to discuss the problem and explain again if necessary. Even the novice rider should be aware if the horse is inclined to drift when it jumps and this should be taken into consideration when choosing the line to the fence and the spot to jump. Correction of these horses should be made when schooling on the flat or jumping in the manege, but many horses never stay quite straight over a fence. Whether they can be corrected depends on why the horse drifts.

- It may be a habit that stemmed from some form of discomfort; even a rubbing brushing boot will make the horse try to land on the opposite leg which will immediately compromise straightness.
- Clearly any history of leg or foot trouble will affect the horse's straightness.
- Commonly any pain or discomfort in the muscles of the back and hind-quarters can lead to a dramatic loss of straightness.
- If the horse has a sore mouth due to sharp teeth or damage inflicted by the bit it will not stay straight.

Horse care is often inextricably linked with performance and both rider and teacher need to be aware of these links. The role of the teacher may involve helping the rider overcome horse care problems in order to enhance performance.

The principles of accurate riding and ensuring that the horse remains in a good quality canter also apply to combination fences where the rider has to choose the line that is best suited to his or her own particular horse. For example, a common 'choice fence' is one that offers a corner, bounce or one stride alternative (Fig. 9.10). Almost every rider would have a preferred route depending on the horse they are riding. However, when riding in competition other factors are brought into play such as time and direction. This means that when developing the rider it makes good sense to encourage the rider to become competent and confident in all three choices. If the rails are straight this does not pose too much of a problem, but if the rails are angled it is much easier for the horse to become confused. The rider must be taught to approach the fence:

- with plenty of confidence;
- in a firm controlled canter;
- on course for the chosen spot;
- keeping the horse straight between the elements;

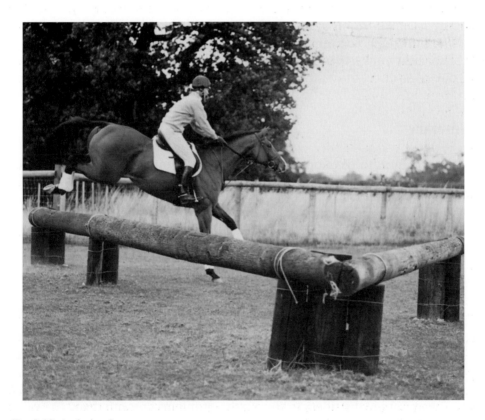

Fig. 9.10 A choice fence.

- keeping in balance;
- with a light elastic rein contact;
- with a secure and encouraging lower leg.

Preparation for competition

Once the riders have schooled over a variety of fences they can start to link them together in preparation for competition. Initially the fences should be on even terrain before progressing to include fences up- and downhill. It is vital to pay equal attention to all the components of successful cross-country riding:

- The approach must be straight and accurate.
- The canter must be the correct tempo, rhythm and balance for the type of fence.
- The rider's position must be adapted to suit the obstacle.
- The horse must be rebalanced as quickly as possible on landing.
- The canter must be re-established and maintained between fences with due regard to terrain, the going and the siting of the next obstacle.

Summary

- Overall aim: to develop the rider's ability to ride over obstacles of all kinds across country and to develop knowledge and understanding of the problems set by nature and man.
- By developing
    discipline
    observation skills
    feel for the effect of terrain, going and the challenge set by the
      obstacles
    self-confidence and thus the ability to overcome fear
    knowledge of the physical demands made on horse and rider.
- Method
    further developing and linking the skills learned earlier to maintain
      the best possible balance, tempo and rhythm at all times and in all
      situations
    encouraging the riders to size up the problems presented and to evalu-
      ate their own and their horses' likely reactions

    progressively introducing cross-country obstacles to ensure confidence
       and ability to remain positive throughout
    developing the feel for riding over a series of fences in preparation for
       competition.
- Lesson management
    mounted or dismounted
    choice of venue
    structuring a series of cross-country lessons.
- Likely problems
    fear of the unknown
    rider losing balance
    rider failing to maintain sufficient impulsion
    rider failing to ride accurate lines
    rider failing to control the horse and thus not able to ride effectively
    lack of access to cross-country facilities.

10   Riding a Course

The rider has already been taught to link together fences indoors, outdoors and cross-country. The next step is to put these skills together to enable the rider to ride simple courses for training purposes, examination and competition. In order to do this the teacher needs to develop the rider's ability to walk and understand distances.

Measuring the distances

Ideally throughout their early training riders should be encouraged by their teacher to ask questions about thez distances and to stride them out for themselves in order to develop a feel for measurement. It is recommended that riders develop the ability to stride accurately either 1 yd or 1 m. (I am 5 ft 6 in (167 cm) tall and of average build and can stride 1 yd to within an inch; however I tried to extend my stride to 1 m and failed miserably!) Initially riders should take three or four active strides and measure the distance that each stride covers. They will then know how much they will have to alter their natural stride in order to pace the distance between two obstacles accurately. Get your students to practise walking distance with their eyes shut and to walk distances alongside you to give them confidence. Novice riders should know the distances for a bounce up to four non-jumping strides between fences, measured from the back of the first obstacle to the front of the next. The only exception to this is if one of the fences is a hog's back, triple bar or pheasant feeder-type fence when the distance should be measured from the middle of the spread fence.

Assuming that the rider has a stride length of 3 ft (1 yd) and that the average competition distance allowing one non-jumping stride between two fences is 24 ft (7.3 m), eight of the rider's strides would indicate an average distance. If there were only seven strides between the fences the distance would be short while nine strides would be a long distance. An easy way to develop this measuring technique is to use Table 10.1.

Table 10.1 Average striding distances.

Feet	Metres	Human strides	Horse strides
24	7.3	8	1
36	11	12	2
45	13.7	15	3
48	14.6	16	3
57	17.3	19	4
60	18	20	4

Different distances can still indicate the same number of horse strides (as shown in the table for three and four horse strides); it is simply a matter of realising that some horses will take shorter strides than others. The implications of this for the teacher are that the rider must become aware of each individual horse's ability to lengthen or shorten its stride while still being able to clear the fence. Table 10.1 indicates that the 'ideal' length of the horse's non-jumping stride between obstacles can vary by up to 3 ft (0.9 m), making a 'long' or 'short' three- or four-stride distance. Its natural stride can be increased or diminished simply by increasing or decreasing the 'revs' and reacting with the correct body balance and rein contact; to some extent the riders have already been encouraged to do this when working over canter poles.

Another way to measure the distance between fences is to allow 6 ft (1.8 m) for landing and 12 ft (3.6 m) for each non-jumping stride between the fences. If you arrive at the next fence with 6 ft (1.8 m) to spare this will be the ideal place for the horse's take-off platform. However, the course designer may lengthen or reduce the distance slightly so that you arrive too far away from or too close to the next fence.

Whichever method is used the important aspect is for the riders to know how many strides they want their horses to take in any given situation.

A training or examination course

Figure 10.1 shows a simple figure-of-eight course which would be ideal for training or examination purposes. It could be changed to add variety and to test different skills of both horse and rider. The suggested track is designed to evaluate the problems of course walking and riding in different circumstances.

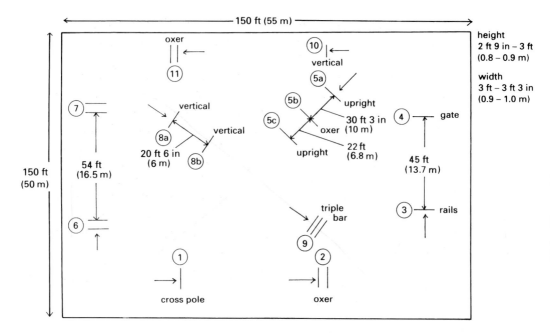

Fig. 10.1 A training or examination course.

Warming up

Fences 1, 10 and 11 in Fig. 10.1 can be used as warm up fences, ensuring steady progression from a cross pole to a vertical to an oxer. Ideally these fences are constructed so that they can be jumped from each rein without having to move poles and fillers. If the rider prefers to start in trot he or she can do so, but the teacher must ensure the quality of the canter before the course is jumped. The importance of the quality of the canter and the strict maintenance of the balanced seat throughout cannot be over-emphasised.

It is a good idea to encourage riders to warm up for this 'course riding' session in the arena amongst the jumps so that they can test the horse's reaction to the fences and other distractions such as vehicles, umbrellas, blowing rubbish, etc. It also gives them a chance to try out the turns that will occur when they are actually jumping. Riders should work in for 15–20 minutes using walk, rising trot, light seat canter, turns, circles and checking the horse's responsiveness to the aids through transitions. The teacher should then introduce the cross pole in trot or canter. As there are other fences in the arena the riders must have thought about where they are going, both on the approach and the landing. The line or track they are going to follow should be one that encourages the horse to stay in balance and rhythm.

The riders can now progress to the warm up vertical at 2ft 9in (0.8m). They should be encouraged to concentrate on the canter rhythm by counting aloud on the way to the fence and resuming counting on landing to help them maintain the same rhythm and tempo. The teacher should try to keep all the riders on the move, allowing them to jump the fence twice and then walking. Obviously they should 'come again' if the jump has not been satisfactory. This should be done on both reins. The riders can now move on to the oxer. To encourage rider confidence this should initially be an ascending spread with the back rail up to 3ft (0.9m) high. The emphasis should be on an upbeat canter with plenty of energy but not too fast, approximately 11 miles per hour (320m per minute).

After the warm up the riders should be asked to consider how they anticipate that the course will ride for them. The riders will have walked the course and should have paid attention to:

- the distances in the double and the combination;
- the related distances;
- the track, i.e. the line from one fence to another;
- the fillers – will they 'spook' the horse?
- are there any turns which may pose a problem?
- where will a change of lead be necessary?
- will the horse hang towards the collecting ring or stables?

For each horse and rider combination the teacher needs to consider:

- the distances;
- will the horse need to be kept energetic?
- will the horse need to be kept calm?
- will the horse need to be pushed on for three strides or will it need to be contained?

The jumps should all be well within the riders' capabilities which should enable them to concentrate on these finer points.

Use of the whip

If the rider anticipates that the horse is likely to spook he or she should know how to deal with this. The rider may simply increase the leg pressure as the horse is turned into the fence. Alternatively if the horse is a slow reacting, lethargic type the rider may give it a slap down the shoulder with the whip. The whip is simply an aid to back-up the rider's leg; however, there may be times when the whip is used to reprimand a horse, for example if it refuses to jump a fence. In these cases the whip should be used with discretion and must never leave a mark on the horse (see Appendix 1).

Riders have two main options for using the whip effectively. Firstly, the whip can be used down the horse's shoulder to attract its attention, but this should not be done within the last three strides before a fence or it may actually distract the horse from the task in hand. The rider must be careful that the horse does not veer away from the whip. If the horse has a tendency to run right then the whip should be in the right hand and vice versa. Secondly, if the horse refuses for no apparent reason it should be turned slightly away from the fence and, with the reins in one hand, given one or two sharp slaps behind the rider's leg and then represented to the fence. It is not advisable to stand the horse in front of the fence and then hit it because:

- the rider cannot allow the horse to go forwards, which is the whole idea of using the whip; and
- it is not permitted under the rules of show jumping as it constitutes showing the horse the fence.

At this stage it is not recommended that the rider takes the hand off the rein on the way to a fence in order to use the whip. Nor is it recommended that the novice rider wears spurs. Riders should learn to be effective without spurs and only use them when they are thoroughly competent and in control of their aids. The whip should be specifically designed for jumping, with a broad, flat end which will reduce the chances of marking the horse. Long dressage whips should only be used by very experienced riders to help with a specific schooling problem.

Change of lead

Before the riders attempt to jump a course the teacher will have encouraged them to be confident in riding a change of rein with a change of lead using a few steps of trot. It is now time for the teacher to consider how the leg on which the horse lands can be influenced even at this early stage in rider education. The most simple approach is for the rider to look in the direction of the next turn. If, for example, the rider is jumping a cross pole on the left rein and wishes to circle left, the rider should look left as the horse begins its descent; this may be enough to ensure that the rider's weight is distributed so that the horse lands on the correct lead. If this fails and the teacher feels that the pupil is sufficiently progressed the rider can open the inside rein to encourage the correct lead on landing (Fig. 10.2). Some horses will always land on one leg and with older horses it may be difficult, if not impossible, to correct. In these cases the rider must decide on the best moment to effect the change of lead through trot. The horse must be allowed to get away from the fence, but the transition must not be left so long that there is not sufficient time to re-establish canter before the next fence.

A good exercise for raising rider awareness of landing on the correct lead is to ask the riders to shout out which leg the horse is leading on as soon as they know after landing over the fence. Later on they can do this with their eyes closed, providing that there are no obstacles in the way. This can first be

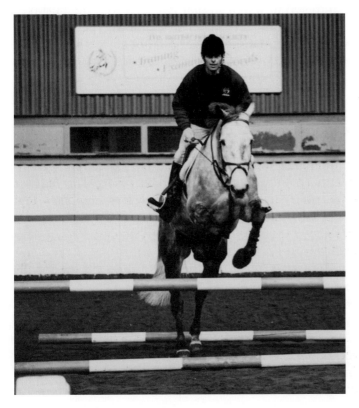

Fig. 10.2 Opening the inside rein.

done in the manege by asking the riders to turn down the centre line, close their eyes and ask for canter, call out the lead and turn in the appropriate direction. The exercise is fun, improves the canter aids and the other riders can join in by observing each other. This is an exercise where placing the riders in a line and each rider performing individually has benefits as the teacher can nominate one of the other riders to check that the rider demonstrating is giving correct information. It is also safer to only have one horse out at a time.

Jumping the course

While one rider is jumping the course the other riders can be either outside the arena, keeping their horses on the move and yet able to observe the other rider, or standing in corners of the arena, turned in to face the jumps. If the horse and rider have been standing they should be given time to walk and canter on each rein before jumping the course. It is important that riders not performing are encouraged to watch so that they can spot the mistakes and see what works well so that they can build it into their own performance. The instructor must take care that the same person is not always asked to be the trail blazer; being the first to go is useful in developing self-belief and confidence.

Evaluating rider response

Even at this stage of rider development riders should be encouraged to prepare themselves mentally for what they are about to do. The teacher should try to encourage riders to evaluate for themselves how they feel about the task ahead. For example:

- Are they confident?
- Do they feel they cannot wait to get out there and show off their skills and impress the instructor and the other riders?
- Do they want to short-circuit the preparation and get on with it?
- Are they nervous?

Some may be good competition riders if they can become sufficiently disciplined and have a natural flair for jumping. There is no doubt that from the start some riders are able to present a horse in balance to a fence; to have such a rider to teach is a richly rewarding experience, but unfortunately it does not happen very often!

Nerves may be due to a fear of falling off or, more commonly, of making a fool of themselves. Riders must be aware that we all learn from our mistakes and part of the teacher's remit is to challenge the riders – to set them problems as well as to help them solve problems. When the worst happens and you are laughed at, somehow it is never as bad as you had anticipated. Perhaps there are times when the teacher has experienced this and can empathise with the rider. Once I was teaching a class of students to long rein in and out of some small jumps, including some work over trotting poles. One student, a tall, well-built young man long reining a tall well-built horse, set off over the poles with a most impressive big trot. Unfortunately the horse caught a toe on a pole, the rider lost his balance and the horse set off in canter towards a small jump. The student made a valiant effort to jump the jump after the horse, failed, somersaulted through the long reins and ended up sitting in the middle of the arena shaking with laughter. All forms of activity involving horses are risky but are also great fun and should be kept so.

The most difficult pupil is the one who takes the whole thing deadly seriously. Such pupils are very hard on themselves when they make a mistake, especially if it is in front of their peers. They must be taught to evaluate their performance positively; no performance can be all bad. We tend to be taught that the horse is never wrong and that mistakes are always the rider's fault. I would dispute this; certainly let the rider evaluate their own performance first, but there are occasions when despite all the rider's skill and correct technique the jump will be knocked down.

The effects of a negative response by the rider to a challenge may include the following:

- Technical skills can break down due to excessive competitive anxiety. For some riders just jumping a simple course under examination conditions is equivalent to an international rider competing in an important Grand Prix. This lack of self-confidence can disturb the rider's concentration on the vital aspects of jumping, namely balance, rhythm and tempo.
- Physical proficiency as muscle tension increases, leading to heaviness of the limbs and a consequent lack of ability to maintain the balanced

supple seat. This can result in the rider giving up both mentally and physically and thus no longer trying.
- The rider is then so confused that the decisions made prior to walking the course are not carried out effectively. Inefficient mistake management skills can then have a subsequent effect of complete loss of the situation, jumping the wrong course as an extreme example or simply missing the line to a fence.

The instructor's role

The instructor needs to develop the ability to improve the rider's skill development in three areas: technical, physical and tactical. During practice the instructor might see the pupil performing well technically, physically and tactically; however, the pupil may not excel in competition. Practice is less stressful and allows the rider to achieve the optimum mental state for success. This in turn begins to prepare those who may be serious competitors later.

The key skills that instructors would like their riders to develop are:

- self-confidence – whatever the challenge;
- calmness – even when under pressure;
- concentration – the rider cannot afford to be distracted;
- discovery of the rider's 'optimal performance state'; this will only become natural when the mental skills allow it to do so;
- mental preparation – for managing mistakes, coping with frustration and snatching opportunities;
- ability to cope with pressure – pressure is the worst enemy of concentration; develop routines and regimes that diffuse pressure;
- ability to cope with stress – coping with the rough and the smooth, the winning and the losing;
- mental skill development by integrating technical, physical and tactical demands leads to the motivation without which even the most simple tasks are impossible.

This theme will be developed further in later chapters on competition training and performance.

After jumping the course, self-evaluation and instructor observations it is often beneficial to repeat the performance. In order to keep all the horses and riders involved it may be better to debrief at the end of all performances rather than after each one. Then the key area to be improved can be identified, a new warm up can take place and the process repeated.

Normally in training sessions and examinations there is more than one opportunity for the riders to show their best performance. Even clear round jumping competitions give the rider the chance to have more than one go. The teacher must ensure that even small improvements are noted and praised; improvement is always valuable and perfection is rarely attainable.

Cross-country courses

Walking the cross-country course effectively is a crucial aspect of successful cross-country riding at any level. Initially novice riders should be encouraged to walk one or two courses with their regular instructor. There may be a formal start box or merely a start point if it is a training course or an examination. The riders should project their minds forward to the first fence; it may just be a simple log but it will mean leaving the other horses behind and going alone. The horse must be thinking forwards and straight with sufficient energy to make the jump easy. For schooling purposes the canter should be about 15 miles per hour (450m per minute). This means that the horse must start positively but smoothly; riders should never be encouraged to jump out of the start like flat race horses leaving the stalls. The horse needs to be calm and the rider should progressively build up to a canter that can be sustained with reasonable ease throughout the course.

Once the first fence has been negotiated the rider must look ahead to see where the best line to the next fence lies. The principles followed during the training sessions must be kept in mind:

- the nature of the fence
    straightforward, e.g. logs, hedges, pheasant feeders
    verticals, e.g. gates, post and rails, walls
    spreads, e.g. ditch and hedge, water ditches, triple bars
    oxers, e.g. hedges with rails, parallel bars, tables
    uphill and downhill fences
    drop fences, into light or dark
    hazards, e.g. water

combinations, e.g. steps, coffins, alternatives
accuracy fences, e.g. corners, arrowheads
- the lie of the land
  flat
  uphill
  downhill
  ridge and furrow
- the going
  hard
  soft
  good
  variable
  stony.

These have all been practised individually and in small groups so the riders should feel confident that they can tackle a short small course in fair conditions. Ideally the course will be half to three-quarters of a mile long (800–1200m) with fences not exceeding 3ft (0.9m) to be covered at a speed of about 15 miles per hour (450m per minute). The rider's first course should not be too long because the mental stress of riding a course will lead to increased physical stress and the rider must be able to keep the horse in balance with sufficient energy. The rider must also be able to maintain his or her balance and influence on the horse until the horse has been pulled up; the rider will not be able to do this if tired.

While walking the course the teacher should involve the riders in the decision making at each fence. One person should not be allowed to take over and the key factors must be covered at each fence:

- the line of approach – accuracy;
- the type of canter – strong or controlled?
- the siting of the fence – light to dark, on the flat or uphill?
- the going – slippery, deep or perfect?
- the relationship of the fence to the one before it and the one after it;
- the position of the fence in relation to the start, finish or lorry park;
- potential distractions;
- the action to be taken if a mistake is made, e.g. taking the alternative;
- will the time of day affect the fence, e.g. sun in the rider's eyes; will the going be cut up if a lot of horses have already jumped?

Pulling up

The teacher must emphasise to the rider the necessity of keeping the horse balanced, straight and on the bit when stopping. The horse should be slowed down as gradually as possible as this is best for the horse in recovery terms and will also reduce the risk of injury to tired limbs. Although these points may not seem relevant over a short training course, it is important to instil good practice from the outset so that it becomes habitual.

Having evaluated the course as a group, encourage each rider to rehearse the fences, the numbers and any special requirements for each one. The riders should know exactly what is coming next and how they are going to cope with each challenge. This positive approach is of great value if the riders decide to go on to compete. Rarely should the rider set out to ride a cross-country course 'playing it by ear'. Although the feel of the horse and the way it jumps may lead to a change of strategy, this is unlikely to be a factor in the early training of the novice rider.

Warming up and the practice fence

The horse and rider need to be sufficiently warmed up – 15 to 20 minutes' walk, trot and canter, followed by four to six jumps over the practice fence should be adequate. There is normally only one practice fence. The riders should start at a speed at which they feel confident, normally a show jumping type canter. They can then progress to building up the canter to a swinging cross-country pace as their confidence grows. If the course demands a fence to be jumped on the angle, this can be practised, but the rider must not get too ambitious. The horse and rider could start brimming with confidence so taking risks at the practice fence is not normally justifiable.

The debrief

After the cross-country session all the riders can be debriefed together so that they can share their experiences. A positive approach should be encouraged by asking for the good aspects before considering the areas that need further training. If other people have had an opportunity to watch, their contribution to the discussion can be useful, while video cameras are an invaluable aid to training. Photographs are useful but are not instantly available. The really important aspect of the training session is that all the riders feel that they have achieved something and have enjoyed their training.

Summary

- Overall aim: to develop the rider's ability to ride a course of fences both show jumping and cross-country; to develop the rider's knowledge and understanding of the challenges offered.
- By developing:
  observation skills
  confidence through mental rehearsal
  the link between the training sessions and riding the course
  interaction between the instructor and pupil and between peers
  feel for the horse through sustained effort.
- Method
  linking knowledge of distances to practical evaluation of each individual challenge set
  rising to meet the challenge of individual performance
  introducing the concept of mental rehearsal and that the rider's state of mind is reflected in performance
  transferring skills to early competition-type experiences.
- Lesson management
  lessons mainly student led
  performance evaluated
  riders supported by peers
  control of groups and awareness of preparation.

11 Advanced Development of the Rider

By now the rider is competent at a level approximately equivalent to the standard required for the British Horse Society Stage III riding examination, in other words he or she is able to compete at a basic level over fences up to 3 ft 3 in (1 m). The rider is now ready to refine the skills learnt in order to enable him or her to become sufficiently educated to train a horse him or herself. In order to train a horse the rider's seat must be totally secure and the rider must be able to adapt his or her balance to suit a variety of horses in a range of different circumstances. How does the teacher go about helping the rider consolidate the security of the seat?

Lunge lessons

The instructor can improve the jumping rider's seat on the lunge provided that the horse is well balanced and accustomed to the work and that the surface being worked on is secure. The instructor must be acutely aware of the centrifugal force involved in lungeing, in other words the tendency of the rider to lean out to counteract the inward pull of the circular movement. Obviously the faster the horse goes, especially if jumping, the greater this tendency becomes; thus the instructor must keep the circle as large as possible. It goes without saying that the instructor should be thoroughly experienced in lungeing a horse over fences before attempting to lunge both horse and rider over fences.

Care must be taken in the selection of the obstacles to be used as it is imperative that there is no chance of the lunge line getting hooked up on a jump wing or cup during the exercise (Fig. 11.1). Bloks are useful for raised trotting poles and small fences, but if they are stacked on each other to make a higher fence they tend to be rather unstable. Jumpkins, synthetic pyramid-shaped wing and tubular steel fences especially created for lungeing, are ideal. Poles should be a standard length (12 ft, 3.7 m) and standard diameter.

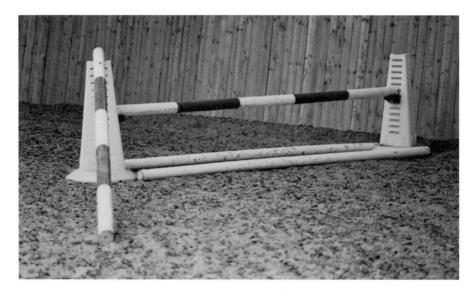

Fig. 11.1 A suitable fence for lungeing over.

The horse should wear a snaffle bridle, neck strap, close contact jumping saddle and brushing boots all round with the lunge rein attached to the lunge cavesson, not the bridle. It should have been warmed up for 5–10 minutes prior to the lesson; this may simply be on the lunge without the rider or ridden off the lunge in the school. The rider should be warmed up with the stirrups at jumping length on a 15 m circle in rising trot and light seat canter. The rider should start with both reins and stirrups while the instructor conducts a 5 minute revision of the correct seat and balance. The range of exercises that could be used is very large and only a few key exercises are outlined here.

Throughout all the exercises the instructor should pay close attention to the detail of the rider's position.

Lesson 1 – improving balance and trotting poles
Once the rider is warmed up the reins can be knotted and tucked under the neck strap. Riding in all three paces the rider can then be encouraged to improve his or her balance by stretching the arms out horizontally, then forward, then down towards the horse's mouth. Attention must be paid to the maintenance of the lower leg position, the rider's back must remain flat while the hips are supple enough to allow the arm exercises to be carried out. The instructor should be in control of the horse, but it is often beneficial for

the rider to use the legs or seat to influence the impulsion as it is very counter-productive if the instructor has to chase the horse with the whip. Should the horse misbehave and buck or try to run off, naturally the rider should take up the reins and impose some control.

Once the rider is comfortable without reins, the instructor can introduce three trotting poles on the circle at the normal schooling distance of 4 ft 6 in (1.37 m) measured to the centre of each pole. The poles should be placed where the jump is going to be, near to the wall or fence, as you should always be lungeing in a safe, enclosed area. The rider should trot in the 'poised' position with the hands forward all the way around the circle and over the poles two or three times while the instructor checks the balance. The rider can then have a break as it is very tiring to maintain this position. The instructor should also check that the stirrups are the correct length to give the rider maximum support. The rider can then be asked to vary the position of the upper body: more upright, more forward, seat light, seat close or seat down. The instructor should observe the rider and discuss with him or her the effects of the different positions on the rider's balance and security. The rein should be changed every 5 minutes. The rider can then progress to trotting over poles raised 4 in (10 cm) off the ground to create more movement for him or her to cope with. The distance between the poles should remain the same. Bloks are ideal for this. Square-ended cavaletti that will not roll can also be used.

This may be all that there is time to fit into the first lunge lesson as 20–30 minutes is ample, including discussions and rests. If the rider or the horse is made stiff or sore they will not benefit from the work.

Lesson 2 – jumping a cross pole and vertical

In the next lunge lesson the rider should be ready to jump a cross pole at about 2 ft 6 in (0.8 m) in the centre. The use of a run-up pole is recommended to help the rider see the line to the fence and ensure that the horse does not run out. Whether or not a placing pole is used largely depends on the horse that is being used. Left to their own devices most horses will find a suitable take-off platform without the assistance of a pole, but if they are erratic then a pole placed 8 ft (2.4 m) away is helpful. A pole on the ground 2 ft (0.6 m) either side of the fence creates the opportunity for the horse to bascule and thus to increase the rider's feel.

Once horse and rider are warmed up as before, the rider can knot the reins but leave them loose on the neck so that the horse is totally free from restriction. The rider must be aware that it is his or her responsibility that the reins are not lost up the horse's neck. Initially the rider should be encouraged to just place each hand on either side of the neck and simply follow the movement. The instructor should keep the horse in trot on the approach and quietly bring the horse back to trot after the fence, with help from the rider if necessary. This should be repeated two or three times on each rein before introducing a small (3 ft, 0.9 m) vertical and progressing to canter. As with previous exercises the rider can be encouraged to count the rhythm to ensure a smooth jump. Then, as with the trotting poles, the rider can vary the upper body position and then the hand position: hands up on top of the crest, towards the mouth or on the shoulder. At all times the rider should be encouraged to feed back how this affects the horse; each horse will probably react differently.

Lesson 3 – jumping a spread

By now the rider could progress to jumping a spread fence. The lesson would comprise of the warm up and then jumping a small cross pole. This can then be converted into a spread by putting a rail behind it at around 3 ft (0.9 m) high with about 3 ft (0.9 m) spread. The rider should be warned that the horse may jump bigger and may be inclined to buck or shoot off on landing. The approach should be in canter with the instructor taking great care, as in all these exercises, that the horse is given adequate room on the approach and that the instructor moves sufficiently quickly through the jump to cause minimum disruption to the rhythm and flow of the canter. After two or three jumps a change of rein should be made and a small parallel (3 ft, 0.9 m) introduced. Poles on the ground in front and behind the fence can be used to encourage the horse to bascule and give it an easy take-off platform.

Once the rider is quite secure and confident these small jumps can be negotiated a few times without stirrups; however, this exercise should only be used occasionally as it can lead to excessive tightening of the knee and the rider being too heavy in the saddle. It is good practice for the emergency situations which may occur when competing.

It is not recommended that horse and rider are lunged over a series of fences. It is more beneficial to have the horse off the lunge for this next stage of the position consolidation work.

Work off the lunge

To encourage the rider to trust the horse it is a useful and fun exercise for the rider to knot the reins and ride the horse round the manege. The rein should be knotted so that the rider can work the horse normally, but if the reins are dropped on the neck there should be no danger of the horse putting its foot in them. For this work the horse would wear its normal jumping equipment plus a neck strap if a martingale is not worn. The exercise can be carried out with a class as well as with an individual and the majority of horses are very co-operative.

Riding down a grid with no reins (Figs 11.2 and 11.3)

The instructor should have the grid already set up with the poles lying to one side ready to put up the fences. The grid might simply be placing pole (8 ft, 2.4 m) to cross pole, one stride (18 ft, 5.5 m) to a vertical, two strides (30 ft, 9.1 m) to a parallel and three strides (42 ft, 12.8 m) to a vertical, set at normal schooling distances, with the jumps 3–3 ft 3 in (0.9–1 m).

The horse and rider should be warmed up and then starting with just one fence the rider should approach the fence in trot and two or three strides

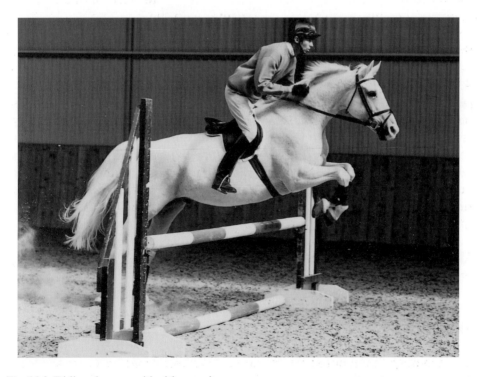

Fig. 11.2 Riding down a grid with no reins.

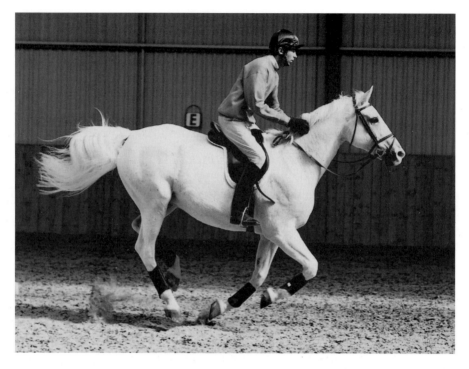

Fig. 11.3 Maintaining the balance between elements without reins.

away put down the reins, place the hands in the jumping position and then pick the reins up again one or two strides after landing. As the rider's confidence grows more fences can be added until the whole grid can be completed. Once the rider is proficient and confident in this, a bounce can be added at the start of the grid. It is remarkable how rarely horses rush or run out during this exercise. A confident instructor with a competent rider can actually do this exercise in the open.

Shortening and lengthening the stride

It is now time to start to educate the rider how and when to influence the horse. One way to start this is to teach the rider to shorten and lengthen the horse's stride over a given distance. During cross-country riding there are times when the rider needs to make the upper body a little more upright in order to contain the horse. At the same time time it may be necessary to do the jumping equivalent of a half halt, but great care must be taken that the rein aid is not too strong, causing the horse to resist the bit, tighten and hollow, thus having a detrimental effect on the horse's jump.

To work over a distance that could be ridden in four or five strides the instructor needs simply to build an upright 3ft 6in–3ft 8in (1.05–1.1m) high to an upright the same height on a distance of 64ft (19.5m). The rider should be able to identify the horse's own normal jumping canter stride and then decide on the action to be taken. For example, if the horse has an average length of stride then the approach to the fence could be as normal; then on landing the rider contains the first stride to make it shorter. Provided the rider maintains a contained canter for the next four strides the horse should be able to put in five strides. To enable the horse to negotiate the distance in four strides, the rider should move the horse on a little for the first two strides after landing then keep the horse balanced and 'on the rein' for the next two strides. Ideally the rider should not alter the stride before take-off as this will change the horse's balance and may cause it to hit the fence. If the last stride is shortened the horse may tighten and hollow while if the stride is lengthened the horse may flatten and lose the bascule. Generally speaking it is easier for the rider to learn to shorten and lengthen over a predetermined distance as most of the rest of the time the rider should be staying in the balanced rhythmic canter advocated throughout.

If the rider's horse is long striding then, in addition to shortening on the first landing stride, the stride should also be contained on the way to the fence in order to put in five strides and enable the rider to present the horse on a 'deep spot' to take-off. How the horse is educated to shorten the stride will be discussed later. If the horse is short striding the rider will need to keep the horse coming to the fence in a little stronger rhythm to encourage it to jump in as far as possible. The rider will then need to move the horse on for the first two strides as outlined above. It may take several attempts before the ideal situation is reached for the individual horse involved. When horse and rider are confident over verticals they can progress to:

- ascending oxer to vertical
- vertical to oxer
- oxer to oxer.

This exercise would normally be taught over three- to six-stride distances.

The stride can also be adjusted in a double or combination of one or two strides, but the rider must always ask the horse to put in the correct number of strides in this exercise, never allowing the horse to put in three strides in a two-stride distance. If the rider lacks discipline with his or her horse in this respect it can be a disaster in competition. To this end it is essential that the instructor builds up the introduction of shorter and longer strides progressively in this situation.

For example, the instructor wants to teach the rider to keep the horse short in a one-stride double consisting of a vertical to an ascending oxer (Fig. 11.4). The exercise starts with the distance of 23 ft (7 m) with the fences around 3 ft 3 in–3 ft 6 in (1–1.05 m) in height. The rider should be asked to keep the horse in a contained energetic canter on the approach, on landing sit up but not down into the saddle, keep the contact on the rein containing the stride and then release for the oxer out. The legs should always remain close but may be passive if the situation merits it. The instructor can gradually shorten the distance to about 18 ft (5.5 m) if the horse and rider can cope.

To lengthen a horse through the middle of a one-stride double the instructor should build an ascending oxer to a vertical on a distance of 23 ft (7 m), again at around 3 ft 3 in–3 ft 6 in (1–1.05 m) (Fig. 11.5). The rider can lower the seat towards the saddle and use the legs to create plenty of forward balanced flow. The ascending oxer in should encourage the horse to jump in fluently, the rider should then keep the horse moving forward but not flat to the second fence, and then rebalance on landing. The instructor can gradually increase the distance up to 28 ft (8.5 m) if the horse and rider are happy with this.

Throughout these lengthening and shortening exercises it is vital that the rider is encouraged to keep counting the rhythm and the strides, to feed back on how he or she feels the horse is responding and, most importantly, to say when he or she feels the horse is at its limit.

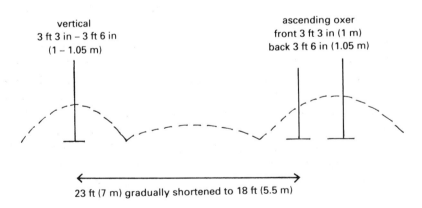

vertical
3 ft 3 in – 3 ft 6 in
(1 – 1.05 m)

ascending oxer
front 3 ft 3 in (1 m)
back 3 ft 6 in (1.05 m)

23 ft (7 m) gradually shortened to 18 ft (5.5 m)

Fig. 11.4 Teaching a horse to shorten through a one-stride double.

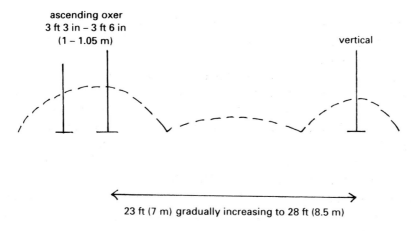

Fig. 11.5 Teaching a horse to lengthen through a one-stride double.

Jumping larger fences

By now the rider should start to jump larger fences. Having worked through the exercises outlined, the rider should be feeling confident about riding related distances. It is natural for the rider to be a little anxious as the fences become larger; the rider is then tempted to try to interfere too much with the horse on the way to the fence in an attempt to get the horse into the right take-off zone. This means that it is probably best to start with an easy three-stride distance of 46 ft (14 m) using an ascending oxer to ascending oxer (Fig. 11.6). This of course must be adjusted if it is not suitable for any reason. The first fence should be kept relatively small (3 ft 6 in, 1.05 m) and the second fence should be gradually built up from 3 ft 9 in (1.15 m) according to the horse's scope.

Once the rider is confident jumping larger fences using this technique, the instructor can then progress to single fences starting with ascending oxers or fences with fillers in front. They can then move onto verticals built from poles at first, progressing on to planks, walls and finally gates. The instructor should keep the emphasis on the rhythm and the balance of the canter and any tendency of the rider to over-check or over-ride should be brought to his or her attention immediately. Any half halt made by the rider should be so subtle that it is almost invisible to the instructor. Equally, 'firing' the horse at the fence needs to be channelled into creating sustained smooth energy within the rhythm.

Jumping larger doubles and combinations should be left until last. Initially

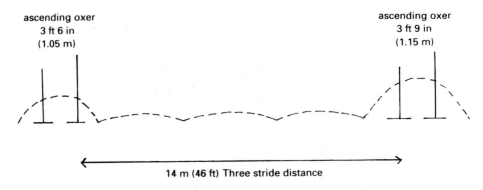

ascending oxer
3 ft 6 in
(1.05 m)

ascending oxer
3 ft 9 in
(1.15 m)

14 m (46 ft) Three stride distance

Fig. 11.6 Using a related distance to introduce a larger fence.

the out fence should be larger than the fence going in to the double; however, the instructor should take care not to build too wide an oxer coming out of a one-stride double, particularly if the rider lacks confidence. The hardest fence for most riders to jump is probably the true oxer, but provided that the canter is good enough and has sufficient energy, then the rider can be encouraged to ride to the fence as if it were a vertical and all will be well. As the rider progresses to larger fences and more complex exercises the instructor must keep a very sharp eye on the rider's position, particularly the lower leg which can lose its security when the horse begins to jump more powerfully (Fig. 11.7). It is hard to put these exercises into an order of priority. They are all equally important and should be incorporated into the training sessions as and when they would be most effective for each individual or group.

The flying change and landing on the appropriate leg

One other vital component in the training and riding of the show jumper is the flying change. A horse that is capable of a balanced, fluent change of lead not only saves valuable time in a jump-off, but also can often ensure a clear round. The rider will have noticed that when the horse is disunited as they approach a fence, because it has changed lead in front but not behind, it is often so out of balance that the fence is knocked down. Equally, if the horse comes round the corner on the wrong lead it may fall out through the shoulder, lose its balance and again hit the fence.

The jumping rider should understand the classical aids for the flying change. The basic principles are those for the canter aid, so that the inside

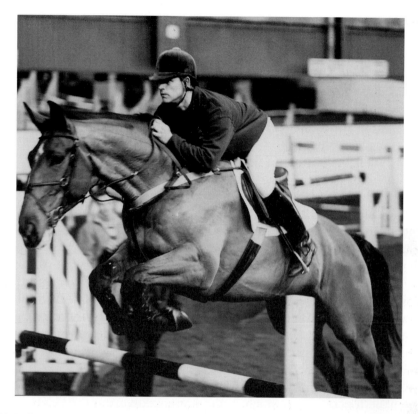

Fig. 11.7 The trainer must keep a sharp eye on the rider's position, especially the lower leg.

leg is supportive and maintains the energy while the outside leg gives the actual signal. If the horse can be kept relatively straight during the flying change this will help the balance. The rider should try to keep the weight as even as possible in the saddle, but if the horse is not very refined in its response it may help to keep the weight slightly towards the new leading leg. Certainly the rider should not sit heavily in the saddle. Teaching the horse to do flying changes is discussed in Chapter 13. Until the rider is very confident riding the changes it is probably best for the rider to ask for the change as he or she comes to the bend which starts the new direction.

It is also necessary for the horse to learn to land on the appropriate leg as it comes over the fence. To encourage this the rider should be asked first of all to open the rein to the new side, for example if the rider wants to turn left he or she should open the left rein, look left and keep the weight slightly to the left. A trained horse will quickly recognise these aids and respond. Over time the less experienced horse will respond providing that the rider is consistent in the aids. However, care must be taken that any aids given as the horse is landing do not interfere with the actual jump. For example, there are instances in high class competition when a rider has started the turn too early over the fence and the horse's inside hind leg has caught the rail and the fence has fallen.

Rein release

The rein release emphasises why the instructor must be so insistent right from the outset that the seat is developed to give extreme stability and balance. This enables the more advanced rider to use the reins, his or her legs and body weight independently of each other as the need arises. To develop this further different types of releases of rein contact can be practised. The two main releases referred to are the short release and the long release. Either releases can be along the crest or towards the bit, or in extremes down the shoulder, although this is not commonly recommended. The principle behind these different releases is that different fences require different amounts of rein.

- A vertical fence or shorter distance demands a minimum rein allowance over the fence, just as much as the horse takes from the rider.
- A long release moves the hand further forward for a longer duration to enable the horse to stretch over wide spreads and longer distances.

These exercises are equally useful for the cross-country rider and the show jumper. An excellent exercise for all riders is to practise a variety of ways of influencing the individual horse by the different forms of crest release. This will enable the correct reaction when competing or when training young or unpredictable horses.

Benefits of riding different horses

During the advanced development of the rider he or she should be encouraged to ride a range of horses so that he or she learns to maintain the position and principles whatever the circumstances. Continually riding problem horses or badly trained horses normally leads to a deterioration of style, skill and harmony and therefore should be avoided if possible. Unfortunately many such horses are offered to good riders to 'sort out' and often more available to them for competition riding; it takes great strength of character to turn them away when most riders are desperate for competition experience.

Summary

- Overall aim: to develop further the rider's skills to enable him or her to train a young horse in the future and to enable him or her to compete successfully to further experience.
- By:
    consolidating the security of the seat
    refining the aids to enable shortening and lengthening of stride
    introducing the flying change
    planning the introduction of exercises for each individual.
- Method
    developing the rider through:
    – lunge lessons
    – free jumping with no reins
    – influencing the horse through the approach, the jump, the landing and the getaway
    – awareness of horse response.
- The tools of the trade
    a variety of horses
    a variety of fences
    lungeing skills and equipment.
- Transferring skills
    maintaining the pure principles when moving on
    which skills are applicable to both cross-country and show jumping
    rider suppleness and confidence.
- Likely problems
    fear of jumping larger fences
    anxiety regarding the take-off platform
    the temptation to compete on problem horses or badly trained horses
    lack of availability of sufficient schoolmaster horses.

12 Teaching Examinations

This chapter aims to give some clear guidelines on the requirements of British Horse Society (BHS) teaching examinations. It includes some overall perceptions of how teaching is assessed, the individual requirements at each level and the training and practice that is needed before taking the exam, as well as suggested lesson plans and proposals for lecture demonstrations to enhance teaching technique. The chapter is designed to meet the needs of both the student teacher and his or her trainer.

All potential teachers should first of all study in depth the subject they are going to teach. This study can embrace:

- reading;
- watching videos;
- attending conferences and lecture demonstrations;
- discussion with colleagues and competitors;
- going to shows;
- observing horse and rider techniques at all levels and in all the jumping disciplines.

Only by thoroughly understanding the sport to be coached can the teacher be really effective. The principle is equally true for the trainee instructor for the Preliminary Teaching Test (PTT) and the senior instructor studying for the BHS Fellowship. There is always more to see and more to learn.

If this book is being used in conjunction with *Coaching the Rider*, also by Jane Houghton Brown and published by Blackwell Science, it will be noted that there is some overlap. This is intentional; one of the mainstays of learning, for both horse and rider, is the need for repetition in order for points to be truly absorbed and retained.

Factors that influence learning to jump

- Motivation – why does someone want to learn to jump? It may be to compete, to hunt or simply as a challenge. The wise teacher will try to ascertain why the pupil wants a lesson and what the pupil hopes the outcome will be.

- Age – jumping is a skill that requires suppleness, balance and quick reactions and it is undoubtedly easier to master when young. However, young riders need to have sufficient physical development to enable them to maintain control and balance.

- The frequency of practice – the more practice the better, provided that the correct technique is being practised; bad habits are just as difficult to eradicate as good habits are to acquire.

- Sex – jumping is one of the few sports where men and women compete on equal terms. More girls than boys start riding, there are more female than male candidates in the exam system and there are more women than men competing at National level, yet at World and Olympic levels in both three-day eventing and show jumping there are more successful men than women – why? Are men simply stronger, braver and possessed of a greater 'killer instinct'?

- Availability of good tuition – however great the talent of an individual rider, this needs nurturing and developing. It is interesting to note how countries like Japan have developed as equestrian nations due to a very structured training plan. At the other end of the spectrum, the better tuition the beginner jumper receives, the more secure his or her foundation will be and the better he or she will be able to progress.

- Availability of good horses – a good horse goes hand in hand with good tuition. The better the schoolmaster the more secure and confident the novice rider will be. Equally as the rider's talents emerge, the need for better and more talented horses that are able to be trained thoroughly becomes a focal point.

- Personal learning styles – everyone learns in different ways. This is one reason why the BHS does not encourage stereotypical teaching, but prefers teachers to study their pupils and their horses so that they can teach them accordingly. This complex subject is covered in more detail in *Coaching the Rider*, but, broadly speaking, most people are either 'doers' or 'thinkers'. A few are balanced evenly and are probably the easiest to teach. The 'doers' want to get on and have a go with the minimum of explanation; they would rather try something out and get it wrong. The 'thinkers' want a sound technical explanation before trying something out.

It can be seen from this broad brush outlook on the theory of teaching that there is much more to teaching jumping than simply putting up the jumps, keeping everything safe and making some corrections. Lamentably one often sees this bare minimum being demonstrated in everyday teaching situations and examinations. The successful teacher must be motivated to do more than this.

What makes a good jumping teacher?

- They must be knowledgeable.
- They must be able to inspire even the most unenthusiastic or nervous rider. To do this they must genuinely enjoy teaching.
- They must be open minded and willing to try out new methods and techniques.
- They must be good planners and well organised but sufficiently flexible to meet the current situation.
- They should have sufficient equestrian skills to be able to demonstrate effectively. Obviously it is recognised that not everybody can be a Michel Robert or a Ginny Leng; those individuals who are able to train and to ride successfully in competitions are a very rare breed.
- They must be able to make corrections in a positive manner that is acceptable to the pupil. This means that they must be able to establish a rapport with their pupils and the way in which the voice is used should be encouraging but firm, in order to develop respect.

Above all the teacher must be able to gain the pupils' respect and ensure that the pupils enjoy their lessons and always finish wanting more!

The BHS teaching examinations

The examination candidate needs to know what the examiner is looking for at each level and how this fits into the overall philosophy of teaching jumping.

The Preliminary Teaching Test (PTT)

The PTT is the first of the BHS teaching exams. The examiner is aware that this is the first level and will make some allowance for this. However, he or she will expect a considerable amount of teaching practice to have taken place. This should be under the supervision of a qualified teacher, preferably of Intermediate standard. As a guide it is suggested that all the subjects listed in the *Examination Handbook* (available from the BHS) are taught prior to the exam. Some subjects will blend together and can therefore be covered in one lesson. Lessons taught should include some that last for a commercial length of time, for example, a 30-minute lunge lesson or a 60-minute class lesson. Special exam technique training can come later on.

The examiner will want to see that the lesson is:

- structured
- progressive
- safe
- enjoyable.

The candidate's experience will be demonstrated by his or her confidence, for example, how well he or she organises the class and the jumping equipment. This may mean that the candidate has to consider the examiners – can they hear what is being said during the lesson? In any case in normal everyday work it may be that the instructor supervisor, parents or colleagues need to hear what the teacher is saying to the pupil. The candidate teacher needs to be able to be heard outdoors as well as indoors. The explanations must be clear, the corrections relevant and the exercises chosen suitable. There must be a formal conclusion with feedback to the riders at the end of the lesson. It is only by regular practice that this becomes second nature so that the candidate is able to teach with confidence and authority on the exam day. With reference to the handling of equipment, this may involve the candidate directing another candidate or a helper to position the poles and jumps to suit the lesson plan (Fig. 12.1).

At the PTT level the key factors to keep in mind are:

- Safety – a safe lesson is one that is well organised by a teacher who is alert to potential dangers such as poorly fitting tack, kicking, loss of control by riders, nappy horses, the weather, sudden noises or movements. Safety is all about *awareness*.
- Rapport – establishing a relationship with the rider. If this is a first meeting then it is probably just a stepping stone, but looked at commercially would the rider come back for another lesson by the teacher?
- Planning – the lesson must be structured and progressive. It must have an introduction, a main core and a conclusion. Obviously plans must

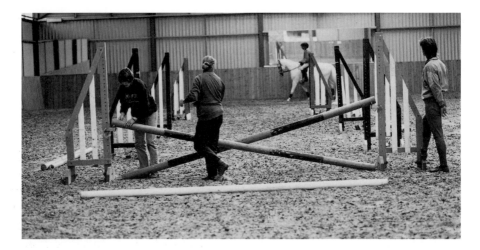

Fig. 12.1 Organising your helper while keeping the rider at work.

be flexible enough to adapt to any situation that the teacher may be in.

* Progression – the candidate must be able to correct the basic faults and establish a basic position from which the riders can jump safely and in balance. In order to do this the candidate's knowledge of the positioning of fences and ground poles must be absolutely secure.
* Pupil involvement – the feedback from the pupil throughout is of paramount importance. This does not mean that the candidate uses the pupil's appraisal of the candidate's own performance in order to opt out of teaching, but it is important to check that the candidate and pupil are in harmony when evaluating the progress towards the chosen goal.

To sum up the key points that the examiner is looking for, the candidate must have the ability to work towards improving his or her pupils' horsemanship, in this case developing the jumping seat and overall balance, security and control. The candidate must teach in such a way that the pupils would return for more lessons, thus making him or herself employable.

PTT lesson plan 1

Brief: assess the riders and work to improve them using work on the flat and over poles and small fences. Time allowed: about 35 minutes.

The ride: four riders, some on ponies that are quite keen, others on horses that are lazy.

Facilities: enclosed area of 20 × 30m minimum. A larger area may have to be shared with another candidate. This will have safety implications and may distract the riders. Three to four fences. Six to ten poles.

Structure of the lesson

The candidate teacher should introduce him or herself to the riders by lining them up with their backs to the examiner. As the tack is being checked, the riders' names should be asked and a little established about them and their partnership with the horse. If remembering names is a problem, write them down with a reference, for example 'Emma, green jumper' or 'Kate, chestnut, martingale'. The teacher should then explain that he or she would like to see the riders work for five minutes in open order on a specified rein so that he or she can assess their current standard and plan the best way forward for the lesson. If the riders are slow to canter they should be encouraged to get going, but the teacher should not interfere except for safety reasons. Assess the riders' balance, control and awareness of each other. This should then be repeated on the other rein before bringing them back and lining them up where the examiner can hear. Each rider should then be asked how he or she felt his or her horse was working and given one or two pointers in readiness for the next session. The candidate should then explain that the format of the lesson is to develop balance and control by using turns, circles and transitions and then progressing to using ground poles to develop jumping position and their ability to jump small fences. It should be explained that it will be necessary to move along quite quickly to achieve this in the given time; thus most of the work will be carried out in trot.

Having chosen the leading file based on observation during the warm up period, the ride should be moved out into closed order, keeping about three-quarters of a horse's length between riders. The candidate should explain the need to circle away and find a new space if the rider is going too quickly, or to cut the corner if being left behind. Initially the ride can be worked on a 15m circle and on the inner track to give the riders control. They should be asked to concentrate on the rhythm, the responsiveness to the leg and the balance through the corners. Each rider should be corrected in turn and praised when some progress is made. After two or three circuits the riders should be asked to change the rein and the exercise repeated. The ride can then be brought forwards to halt and the riders asked to shorten their stirrups. While they are doing this the candidate can ask a helper to put one pole at least 6ft 6in (2m) in from the track on one side of the school and three poles on the other side, 4ft 6in (1.37m) apart, again in from the track.

The riders can then be asked to demonstrate at halt the position they would adopt both over the poles and between the poles (the 'two point position' as discussed in Chapter 6 'Strengthening the position'). If there is a significant difference between the two, the candidate teacher should explain the reasons for maintaining uniformity. The ride can then go out and practise the position using the same exercises as before. The riders should be corrected, with explanations, and the work developed to include jumping over small fences. The correct techniques to use are outlined in Chapter 6.

If time allows the riders should be worked on both reins before concluding the lesson. The ride can either be brought in and lined up or kept walking on a circle for the debrief. Positive feedback can be encouraged by asking a positive question such as, 'Which part of the lesson did you enjoy most?'. The riders' answers can be used to indicate possible areas for homework. If the examiners ask for the lesson to conclude early the candidate must not try to fit everything in in a rush; equally he or she must not stop the lesson dead. The lesson should be brought to a realistic close and the feedback carried out. It is important not to feel pressurised by the time element. As long as the candidate clearly has the enthusiasm and commitment, the examiners will not expect perfection.

PTT lesson plan 2

Brief: assess and work towards improving the riders' work in canter and then over a one non-jumping stride double. Ensure that the lesson works progressively towards jumping a double. Time allowed: about 35 minutes.

It is unlikely that an examiner would select this as the first lesson of the day, so the ride will already be warmed up and ready to progress. The candidate teacher may have observed or assisted at the previous lesson and it is important to have assimilated as much information as possible about the riders.

Structure of the lesson
It is important to progress the lesson as quickly as possible from the outset. As before the candidate should introduce him or herself while checking the tack and finding out about the riders. The riders should be asked to put their stirrups at jumping length and then sent away to show their horses at the

three basic paces with the emphasis on the canter. Initially the ride should be kept on one rein for safety reasons while the candidate assesses the riders. If during these initial observations there are discrepancies in the balance of the riders' seats the candidate should discuss this with them and try to set them on the road towards improvement, before embarking on the main part of the lesson.

As most of this lesson is to be in canter the importance of maintaining the rhythm must be emphasised. This can be done by asking the riders to canter as individuals, counting out the rhythm as they go. If they find this difficult it is the candidate teacher's job to give them guidance and advise them if the tempo needs to go up or down. If the horse finds it difficult to maintain canter then realistic targets should be set, such as just cantering a 20 m circle, to avoid the horse continually falling back into trot.

When each rider has been worked individually on both reins the lesson can proceed towards jumping, starting with one fence. A small upright of about 2 ft 6 in (0.7 m) is usually appropriate. The wings for the next fence should already be in place at around 18 ft (5.5 m) from the first. The cups and poles should be kept safely to the side. The jumps should be positioned off the track and about half-way down the school; this allows enough room to present the horse to the first fence and enough room on landing over the second fence to turn safely. The ride should be kept moving round the school; the horses are athletes and should not be stood in line getting cold and then asked to come out and perform. In this short time it may not be possible to jump off both reins, so the candidate should choose the rein that the majority of the horses seem more comfortable with. The riders should be asked to jump from canter straight away so that the candidate can ascertain how competent the riders are and how much work there is to do.

The candidate can suggest to the ride that today they are going to concentrate on rhythm and balance, and having initially assessed the riders' abilities in these areas the candidate can make corrections to help the riders towards improvement. Avoid giving too much advice on the way to the fence as this can be distracting. However, the riders should be encouraged to evaluate their own performance so that positive goals can be set. Once all the riders have successfully, if not perfectly, negotiated the single fence, the second fence can be added. Each rider should be asked how he or she thinks his or her horse will react and what sort of action he or she may have to take, with the candidate teacher giving advice where necessary. The riders can then jump the double, keeping the same principles in mind as before. The candidate must be prepared to alter the distance and/or the height of the fences if necessary. It is not possible to teach everything in one lesson; choose one or two key points linked to rhythm and balance and build from there.

The candidate should try to choose a finishing point for the lesson when each rider has done the same amount of work. If there is one rider who is much better or much less confident than the others and needs extra individual time try to keep the whole class interested by involving them in the evaluation of what is taking place. If for any reason the candidate has not been able to fulfil the brief he or she should discuss this with the examiner, who will normally be very understanding. As usual at the end of the lesson, the candidate should encourage a positive debrief from the riders so that they go away feeling fulfilled.

The candidate will be expected to be able to discuss his or her teaching techniques, the placing of the fences and heights and distances, showing a positive attitude without being dogmatic. Potential PTT candidates should work their way through the questions in the *Examinations Handbook* and attempt to discuss them in a group situation in order to improve their discussion techniques. This will also check that they have thought out how these questions may be approached from different angles. During the examination the candidates do not have to agree with everyone else in their group, but should be able to make a logical and sensible argument backed up by sound reasoning to explain their point of view.

The Intermediate Teaching Test

In order to take this exam the candidate must be a minimum of 20 years of age with considerable experience of teaching post-PTT Experience of competing and training riders for competition is invaluable, accompanied by extensive study. Although in the exam the candidate is unlikely to be asked to coach a rider over cross-country fences, this is part of the syllabus, and in order to be convincing in discussion this aspect should not be neglected in training. An instructor who has achieved the Intermediate Teaching Test is expected to be capable of training students for the BHS Stage III exam which demands a competent cross-country performance.

There may be two aspects of jump teaching tested: one an individual jumping lesson and the other with a class, either teaching the riders on the flat for 20–25 minutes or building up to a line of fences. Practise at taking a class lesson and either building up to a line of fences or a grid is an integral part of the preparation for the exam. The candidate should be experienced in teaching lessons ranging from 20 to 45 minutes so that he or she is at ease and knows exactly how the lesson plan is going to work out. It is useful to have prepared several plans prior to the exam and, with any luck, one of these plans will suit the class in the exam. The examiner will question the candidate on the lesson content and where he or she would go from there. Any answers may be probed further, so if the candidate talks about grids or specific competitions, he or she must know the correct technical answers.

Candidates should consider how they would cope if there were no fences set up at all, or if the existing line of fences had to be amended. They must be certain about the distances between fences and where they want the fences to be placed (Fig. 12.2). It is easy for the time to run away while the candidate is just getting organised. Unlike the PTT the candidate is much more likely to be working at an unfamiliar centre with unfamiliar equipment and pupils. The examiners are aware of the added pressure this places on the candidate and will be as helpful as possible. If an exercise is already set up, be sure to check that the distances are suitable before asking the pupils to jump. Confirm the exercise and distances with the pupils and ensure that they are happy to perform the exercise. Above all when teaching, especially jumping, choose exercises that are relevant to the individual pupil and situation. As with the PTT candidates should work their way through the expected questions and must feel confident to discuss any aspect of jump training and teaching that may come up.

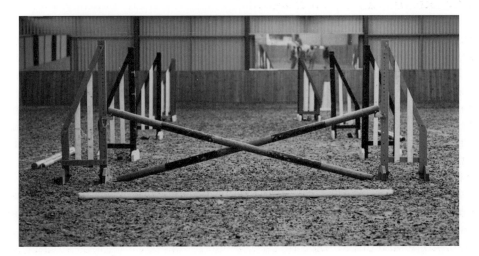

Fig. 12.2 Positioning the wings at the correct distances before starting to use the grid.

Intermediate Teaching Test lesson plan 1

Brief: assess the horse and rider in an individual jumping lesson and work to improve the horse's technique and the rider's influence, using fences in a constructive manner. Time allowed: 35 minutes, to include discussion.

Ideally the pupil will have worked in, but this is not always possible, and the lesson may have to be adjusted on the day depending on the actual pupil available. The candidate is expected to show a sound knowledge of safe procedures, fence construction and of related distances so that he or she can give practical help to riders working towards Newcomers/Novice Horse Trial competitions. Depending on the individual to be taught, the fences should be up to 3 ft 6 in–3 ft 9 in (1.05–1.1 m).

Structure of the lesson

The candidate should first of all find out as much as possible about the pupil, the horse and the pupil's perceived problems. The pupil should then be asked to work in all three paces, with the emphasis on canter. After five or ten minutes, when he or she feels sufficiently warmed up, the rider can be asked to pop over a small fence from trot and canter, off both reins. The fence could be a cross pole or a small vertical at about 2 ft 9 in (0.8 m). Based on the performance over this fence the candidate should then choose appropriate exercises to develop the lesson. The fences should be gradually raised unless a problem develops. Use of all types of ground poles and A-frames is acceptable, providing that the distances are correct for the horse and that the exercises can be justified with clear explanations. As the lesson time is quite short it is not advisable to radically alter the rider's position unless what he or she is doing is clearly detrimental to the horse. If, in the long-term, modification to the rider's position would be beneficial, it should be explained that this would take time to achieve. The greatest care should be taken if the tack is adjusted in any way, for example removing or altering the fit of a martingale. Never do this unless it has the full support of the pupil and the examiner. If for any reason the lesson cannot be progressed because the rider is frightened or the horse unsound, the candidate should discuss with the examiner the best way to continue.

If the candidate feels that the horse requires a considerable amount of work on the flat, he or she should explain that this would take several sessions and would be a longer-term goal. It is important from the examiner's point of view that he or she sees the candidate demonstrating confident and progressive use of the fences.

Some evaluation should be made of each jump; it may be a comment on the approach, take-off, landing or getaway or the horse's technique over the fence. It may be complimentary or constructive criticism, but try never just to say 'come again'. Examinations are all about selling yourself to both the pupil and the examiner. Remember, the examiner wants to see progress towards improvement.

Example lesson
Rider: Emily
Horse: Do Good, 16.2 hh (172 cm), six-year-old Novice event horse with a tendency to rush and get a little flat towards the fences.

Watch the horse and rider warm up and jump a couple of fences in trot and canter. The rider can be seen to be competent but the horse is quite impetuous. Ask the rider if she is happy to work with a placing pole. If she says 'yes', put a pole 8 ft (2.4 m) from a vertical 3 ft (0.9 m) high. Ask the rider to trot to the fence, keeping the horse very quiet, using a fairly short approach and sitting very lightly on the approach. Tell her not to panic if the horse canters the last stride, but just to stay in balance and pull up softly in a light seat on the other side. Watch the rein contact carefully and look for any tendency of the rider to 'fire' the horse at the fence, and act accordingly. The fence should be jumped in this way a couple of times before changing the rein and repeating the exercise. The fence can then be made into a 3 ft (0.9 m) square parallel and the exercise repeated, i.e. approaching in trot, using a placing pole and working on both reins. As soon as the horse improves, reward it and move on to the next exercise. Remember, do not expect perfection, just improvement.

The next step is to jump out of canter. Move the placing pole to 18 ft (5.5 m) away from the jump and explain to the rider that there will be one stride from the pole to the fence. Emphasise the importance of a regular rhythm and keeping the approach short with the rider sitting quietly but keeping the horse in balance. Move the pole if necessary. Increase the height and spread a little and ask the rider to come from both reins until some improvement is shown, always checking with the rider what she is feeling.

Then progress to a three stride related distance of 45 ft (13.7 m), starting with an oxer to an upright about 3 ft 3 in high and using a canter placing pole as before. If the horse rushes between the two fences try a landing pole at 12 ft (3.6 m) after the first jump. This will encourage the horse to shorten the first stride. Check that the rider has not altered the rhythm in any way and is not pushing the horse between the two fences. If she is restraining the horse, how is she doing this and how is the horse reacting? Advise as necessary. If all is going well and the horse is improving either make the second fence an oxer or raise it. The canter pole may be taken away if the rhythm is good. Whichever you decide, finish on a good note and do not be tempted to do too much. Make sure your pupil is certain of what she has done, that she is positive in her outlook and knows what she wants to do between now and her next lesson.

The BHS Instructors (BHSI) examination

This exam cannot be taken until the candidate is 22 years old and it is expected that considerable experience will have been amassed since taking the Intermediate Teaching Test. Potential candidates should grasp every opportunity for the study of jump teaching and training, especially if their daily work involves teaching mainly novices, and the opportunities for teaching at the level required for the exam are limited. Certainly some practice at coaching competition riders is essential, and if this is not available at home it will have to be sought elsewhere, perhaps at one of the BHSI training yards or a competition yard. Candidates are expected to be able to coach effectively up to Intermediate Horse Trials standard, using fences up to 4ft (1.2m) high, including combinations and related distances of three, four and five strides.

The format of the exam is similar to the Intermediate Teaching Test, except that more time is allowed – about 45 minutes. The guinea pig rider will have warmed up and, as before, the candidate will have established the horse and rider's background and future aims. The initial assessment is given to the examiner, describing the horse's:

- temperament
- balance
- rhythm
- acceptance of the aids
- general standard of training.

The horse is then jumped over a fence and the following are assessed:

- approach
- take-off

- technique – shoulders, forearms, use of the neck, hindlimbs
- landing
- getaway.

Based on these assessments a lesson plan is formulated and the examiner retires to watch the progress of the lesson. If the candidate feels that it would be beneficial to ride the horse him or herself this is quite acceptable, but it must be remembered that the aim is to teach the rider to school the horse. As before, any exercises can be used provided they are safe and relevant.

It is not necessary to jump a whole course, but if the rider has specifically asked for help in this area then of course it must be given. It is most likely that another person will be teaching at the same time; the candidate must be aware of this and negotiate the use of the fences so that there is harmony with the other teacher. Safety must also be paramount and the other teacher warned where there could be a clash of direction, for example. There will be helpers to move and put up fences, but the distances and construction of the fences must always be checked. Many potential BHSI candidates find it useful to attend the exam as a helper and/or guinea pig before taking the exam. This enables them to have first-hand experience of what the exam is really like. Further details are available from the BHS Training and Education office.

Summary

- Overall aim: to develop a strategy that will enable the candidate for BHS teaching exams to perform effectively.
- By:
    understanding the exam requirements
    studying the subject thoroughly
    being aware of the needs of pupils and their horses.
- Method
    gaining sufficient teaching experience to be confident
    allowing enough time for study and remaining open-minded whilst still
        having a firm teaching strategy
    studying people and their reactions to training and competition.
- Transferring skills
    of training the horse and rider, both on the flat and over fences, to an
        artificial situation

by having clear plans that are readily adaptable to cope with the situation facing the candidate.

- Likely problems

  nervousness and lack of confidence

  unsuitable pupils or equipment

  lack of sufficient preparation, in terms of practice teaching or study.

PART III

TRAINING THE HORSE AND RIDER

13 Training the Horse on the Flat

Primary requirements

The basic training of the jumper on the flat should be the same as for any other discipline, the primary requirements being to develop:

- responsiveness
- suppleness
- balance,

thus ensuring that the horse's jumping ability can be utilised to its fullest extent. Before going any further it is useful to explore the meaning of these three terms.

Responsiveness is:

- the ability of the horse to go willingly forward when asked to do so and to 'think forward';
- the ability of the horse to yield to the bit and come back when asked with as little resistance as possible;
- the ability of the horse to move away from the leg as required, either laterally or simply to conform to circle aids.

Suppleness is:

- the ability of the horse to develop to a stage where it can flex its joints easily and without tension and stiffening of the muscles which will inhibit the full use of the horse's body and prevent it maximising its potential.

Balance is:

- the ability of the horse to develop the three paces in such a way that it can work in balance at all times and in all situations, in other words that it is in 'self-carriage'.

These three fundamentals can only be developed if the following are present:

- adequate conformation and paces for the job the horse has to do;
- an educated rider who thoroughly understands each phase of training and has a firm but sympathetic approach;
- a reasonable temperament. The trainability of the horse is a vital component; the easier it is to train the more progress can be made.

All horses benefit from a sound beginning and many trainers have their own specialities, for examples some are especially gifted at breaking and starting young horses. At the other end of the scale other trainers are talented competition riders. Those who wish to train horses as a career should look at themselves and discuss with their own trainer their strengths and weaknesses and then set themselves realistic targets.

Assuming that the horse has been well broken and can walk, trot and canter without undue resistance or loss of balance it is ready to train on. It is often beneficial for training riders to see the horse working to enable them to make an evaluation of the horse's current stage of training. This is best done by observing the horse on the lunge and under saddle, being ridden by a competent rider who may be their own trainer. During this evaluation the basic principles must be remembered:

- responsiveness
  - does the horse have to be kicked forwards?
  - does it respond to a light rein aid to stop?
  - how much does it fall in through the corners?
- suppleness
  - does the horse flex its hocks well and step underneath or does it drag its toes?
  - are there any signs of stiffness in the back or neck; do these lead to irregularity?
- balance
  - is the horse naturally well balanced or does it easily fall onto its forehand?
  - is the canter a true three time gait?

These are just a few of the questions that potential horse trainers should ask. If this is the first horse they have trained they will need some help and guidance with this evaluation.

The physical wellbeing of the horse cannot, of course, be overlooked. The horse must:

- be sound, i.e. not lame;
- be fit enough for the demands of the work;
- have teeth and feet in good order;
- have tack that fits properly.

Most horses can start their career in a snaffle bridle, normally with a flash noseband to discourage resistance. The bit would normally have one joint and a loose ring, but if the horse reacts abnormally to this then the trainer needs to understand the range of snaffles and nose bands available and choose something more suitable. A close contact saddle that fits the horse and does not pinch or press anywhere is ideal. If the horse is lively the trainer must not be ashamed to use a neck strap. This is better than hauling on the horse's mouth or, worse still, falling off which undoubtedly frightens the horse just as much as it does the rider.

The aim of the training is to develop the jumping and the flat work hand in hand so that as the horse develops strength and balance it can be encouraged to progress (Fig. 13.1). All of the exercises can be practised in the jumping paddock so that the horse does not always associate that area with jumping. It is very good for the horse's mind to develop the horse's responsiveness whilst working in amongst the jumps; it gives the trainer time to evaluate the horse's attitude to the fences, how it copes with the turns and how easy the horse is to 'move up and down the gearbox'.

If all is progressing well the trainer/rider can move on to enhance further the horse's suppleness and engagement by introducing smaller circles in canter, perhaps using the spiralling exercise discussed in 'changing direction and yielding to the leg' to work down to a 10m circle. Another exercise that works well is to establish a 20m circle and when the balance feels adequate to ride a 10m circle and then to return to the 20m circle.

Developing responsiveness

The horse must go willingly forwards; it should not be necessary to resort to spurs in this early work. Equally the horse must accept the lower leg against its side, the fact that the leg is there, softly, all the time should not deaden the horse; this only happens if the rider constantly flaps the legs in order to get a response. So, if the horse does not move forward at a slight nudge or

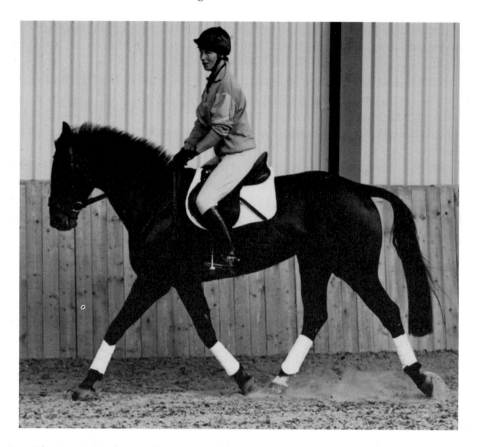

Fig. 13.1 A young horse working confidently on the flat.

squeeze from the rider then this must be backed up by the whip; even with
jumping horses, a dressage schooling whip may be best for this purpose. The
rider's stirrups, however, should not be at dressage length but a multi-
purpose schooling length so that the horse becomes accustomed to an aid
given from a shorter leg. The stirrups should not be so short that the rider
may be dislodged if the horse has a buck and a kick.

Every rider and trainer has opinions on how they would like the horse to
respond and this is perfectly acceptable. Equally each horse will have its own
natural degree of responsiveness that the rider is going to develop. The
responsiveness to the forward aid is enhanced by making transitions. The
frequency and directness of these transitions will vary according to the stage
of training. For example, an inexperienced four-year-old would perhaps
only make three or four transitions around a school of 20 m × 40 m, and

these would be progressive, i.e. trot to canter, whereas a five- or six-year-old may be asked to make a series of transitions over a few strides. Remember, the aim is for the horse to move forward immediately when asked; this may be crucial later when riding to a large spooky oxer. Once the basic principle of moving up a gear is understood then variations within the pace can be introduced, especially at trot and canter. However, it is important that the horse is not allowed to come out of balance during this work. The major difference between schooling the jumper and the dressage horse is that the dressage horse should change in its frame as it lengthens and shortens the strides in order to cope with the movements that are asked, while the jumper needs to keep in as consistent a frame as possible, neither lengthening nor shortening excessively but finding a balance where the strides and the speed can vary without loss of balance or self-carriage.

Responsiveness to the bit

Each horse and rider will vary but in general the jumping horse should not be encouraged to pull; it must accept a comfortable, light, elastic contact which has been generated by the rider's leg. Generally speaking, problems arise with the contact when the horse's conformation is not ideal; for example, if the horse's neck is set low onto the withers it will tend to fall onto the forehand and lean on the bit. Alternatively the horse may work with a naturally high head carriage and an inverted back; these horses tend to run through the bridle and take an inconsistent contact. The key for the rider is to give the horse a consistent contact and to encourage the horse to remain flexible in its jaw by sending subtle signals down the rein whilst pushing the horse forward with the legs. Great care must be taken not to drive the horse aggressively with the seat as this will make it run against the bridle or hollow its back and become resistant. There should never be a situation where the rider sits back and down against the horse and uses his or her weight to pull the horse up. Light aids encourage light response and if this is not taught at the start as the demands increase there can be a tendency for the horse to get stronger and stronger. The use of the voice to soothe and reassure the horse is a useful aid that should not be undervalued.

For very sensitive horses early work in walk – simply walking and halting the horse – in a very undemanding manner can be beneficial for establishing confidence and responsiveness.

The use of training aids such as draw reins should only be resorted to if the horse has an exceptionally difficult temperament or if its conformation makes it very difficult for the horse to accept the aids without fighting. It is desirable to avoid confrontations, and provided that running reins are not used as a means of forcing the horse's head down or as a short cut, they can have a place in the training scheme.

Altering the stride length

The horse must respond to a light aid when making a downwards transition. Once the horse has been worked through the transitions from one pace to another, transitions within the pace can be introduced, mainly in trot and canter. The influence of the rider's body and mind is very important. For example, if the rider is in rising trot and asks the horse to lengthen the steps, the rider will have to incline his or her body a little more forwards in order to stay in balance. However, when the rider wishes to shorten the stride he or she should bring the body a little more upright while still remaining light in the saddle. The same principle applies in canter. The amount of 'push' the horse will need to make a significant difference to the stride will depend on the individual, but the main aim is that the horse:

- keeps its balance;
- continues stepping under with the hind legs;
- has free mobile shoulders.

The rider should not allow the horse to become strung out or excessively deep with the nose behind the vertical. What should the trainer do if the horse does not lengthen but merely goes faster? Firstly the rider should be asked about the horse's natural capacity; if the horse is limited in trot this is not too much of a problem for a jumper, but if the horse cannot alter its canter stride this may become a problem as the work progresses. Exercises that help to develop the stride include:

- the use of trotting poles on the ground. Initially the poles should be placed 4 ft 6 in–5 ft (1.37–1.5 m) apart and gradually moved further apart until the desired length of stride is shown. It is important to use the same driving and restraining aids to obtain the lengthening so that when the poles are removed the horse still understands what is required. The poles can also be raised a few inches off the ground at one or both ends. This is very useful if the horse does not use its hocks or shoulders sufficiently. Generally it is not necessary to both raise and widen the poles – one or other is enough.

- the use of canter poles. A similar exercise can be used in canter, starting off with the poles at about 8–9 ft (2.4–2.7 m) apart and gradually raising them or widening them. A series of six to eight poles placed 9–10 ft (2.7–3 m) apart and about 18 in (45 cm) off the ground is a very effective strengthening and balancing exercise for both horse and rider.

When working with poles it is important that they are secure to give the horse confidence.

At this stage when working the horse to increase responsiveness, the half halt is being brought into play to rebalance the horse before a change of pace or direction. To execute the half halt the rider keeps the legs close to the horse and nudges the horse to alert it. At the same time the rider closes the fingers around the rein, adjusts the body balance and then either allows the horse forwards, indicates a change of direction or takes another feel down the rein to adjust the speed.

Changing direction and yielding to the leg

The horse should always look in the direction it is going and its body should conform to the line it is going to take, so that in effect the horse is straight whether on a circle or a straight line. It is important that the trainer/rider knows how to correct the horse if, for example, it falls onto the inside shoulder through a turn. The rider must ensure that the horse is prepared to move away from the rider's inside leg. The easiest way to teach this to a young horse is on a circle using a simple spiralling exercise. Starting in walk, the size of the circle is gradually decreased to around 10 m; the horse is then asked to increase the circle by moving away from the inside leg used at the girth. This encourages the horse to step out and across with the hind legs. It is important that the horse:

- maintains the rhythm;
- continues to accept the bit softly;
- remains lightly flexed to the inside of the circle.

The rider should:

- control the degree of the yield, i.e. the horse's outside shoulder should always be under control;

- remain straight with the horse, neither slipping in nor out;
- not allow the horse to take over; each step should be under the rider's control.

As with all training the exercise should be performed evenly on both sides. Once the horse has mastered the technique in walk it can build up to trot and canter, but the circles should not be too small in the early stages otherwise the horse will not be able to maintain the rhythm and balance throughout. This exercise helps the horse turn corners in the ring as it will have increased the horse's flexibility and developed the rider's awareness of the horse's stiff or supple side.

Generally when working on changes of direction, each hand should stay on its own side of the neck so that the horse is working down a direct rein. Serpentines and figures-of-eight in trot are extremely beneficial. The exercises should be varied so that the horse does not anticipate. Ideally the work area is also changed, using enclosed spaces, open areas and varying terrain. This is just as important for the show jumper as for the event horse as it develops balance and power.

Before changes of direction in canter are able to be fully developed the horse should be taught the flying change, that is to be able to change the canter lead without returning to walk or trot. Some horses will show early flair for this and offer to change when working out in the field and moving from one direction to another. These are often horses with a good natural adjustable canter, the ideal show jumper. Other horses, especially thoroughbreds, with longer flatter strides have to be taught to change.

The prerequisites for teaching flying changes to the horse are:

- the horse is absolutely clear on the canter aid itself;
- the horse can canter from walk 'on the aid';
- the canter is adjustable and not 'on the forehand';
- the rider has had experience of riding changes on a schoolmaster.

For the show jumper and even the event horse, using a pole on the ground can be a good catalyst to introduce the change. However, the trainer/rider must be aware that the horse will be inclined to jump into the change (Figs 13.2 and 13.3). Thus it is very important that the rider is able to maintain a light balanced seat throughout and simply give a clear positive aid so that when the pole is removed the horse still understands when and where to change. The pole should be positioned in the school or field so that the

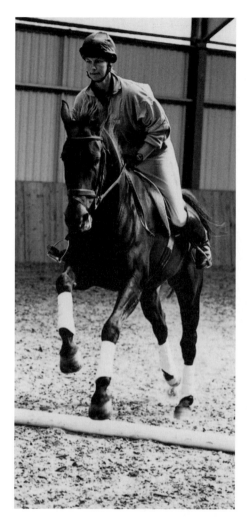

Fig. 13.2 The flying change – note the aid being given by the leg.

change of direction can be made easily without having to inhibit the horse. It may be easier to ask the horse to change from its best canter and only ask for one side for a few sessions before moving onto the more difficult side. Horses will always try to move their bodies to come underneath the rider's weight and this can be used to advantage when educating the young jumper. However, there should not be any violent flinging of the rider's or horse's body onto the new leading leg.

The procedure is to establish as good a canter as possible, check out the line to be taken and make a change through one or two walk or trot strides,

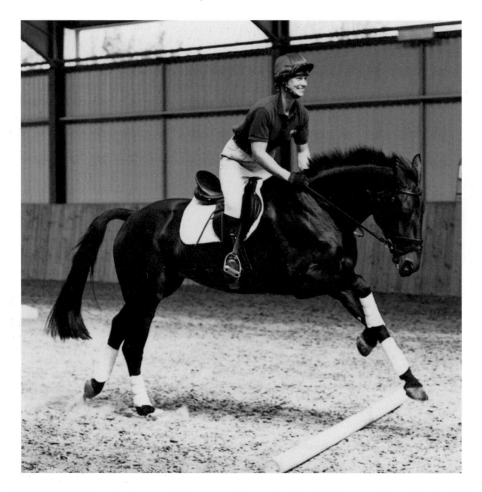

Fig. 13.3 The flying change – note the young horse coming off the ground in order to make the change.

as dictated by the horse's stage of training. Having checked the line and the horse's obedience, the pole should be approached in a good bouncy canter and as the horse bounds over the pole the rider swings the horse into the new direction. Most horses change quite naturally using this method. However, if the horse still does not respond the pole can be raised off the ground to ensure that the horse 'gets off the floor'. The horse should be praised when it achieves the desired result and the exercise should not be repeated more than two or three times on the first few occasions. The rider should guard against the horse becoming excited and strong. The aim is for the horse to change legs naturally and easily to enable it to get from one fence to another with maximum ease.

If the horse is lazy through the change and does not come through with the hind legs a tap with the whip is often most effective. However, the trainer should encourage the rider to be analytical – if the horse is not changing correctly the rider should ask him or herself why this is so. More often than not it is because the quality of the canter is simply not good enough. If this is the case the canter should be checked and repaired. Horses can become quite cheeky when learning changes and start to offer them when they choose rather than on request. The rider should not worry and never scold the horse; it is unlikely to become a long-term problem.

The rein back

One of the most useful engagement exercises is the rein back. This is because, provided the horse steps back from the leg rather than the rein, it encourages the horse to lighten the forehand, thus enabling the horse to step underneath better with the hind legs. It is a good idea to introduce the concept of the rein back fairly early in the horse's training, once the horse accepts the aids for the halt and will stand straight and balanced over all four legs for up to four seconds.

To ask for the rein back the horse should be halted parallel to a wall or hedge. The rider closes both legs behind the girth, but instead of allowing the horse forwards, resists with the rein. As the horse has nowhere else to go it should offer to go backwards. If the horse tries to swing the quarters towards the open side of the school or paddock the horse should just be flexed a little in that direction; this will usually straighten it. As soon as the horse offers to back, even one step, it should be stopped and praised. The horse should never be pulled back. If the horse is unwilling to try, a person on the ground can assist by gently tapping the front legs until it responds. The use of the voice is also very helpful.

Shoulder in

The next engagement exercise could be the shoulder in, that is when the rider asks the horse to take its forehand in from the track whilst the hind legs travel down the straight line, normally describing a 30° angle at this stage of training. The footfalls describe three distinct tracks: right hind, left hind and right fore, and left fore. The horse should look to the left when going to the left and the bend should be softly uniform throughout the body. The hind legs should not cross; this indicates that the movement has degenerated into a leg yield. Ideally the horse should remain in rhythm, continue to accept the bit and stay in balance. The rider must take particular care that the horse does not fall out through the outside shoulder, that is drift out on a corner or circle.

It is easiest to use the corner of the school to set up the movement. The rider should use the rein to position the front of the horse to the in-side. The outside rein controls the pace and regulates the degree of neck bend. The inside leg maintains the energy and bend by staying close to the girth while the outside leg aids the control of the outside of the horse. The rider's body should be turned slightly to stay parallel with the horse's shoulders. It is often best to introduce the shoulder in in walk until the horse understands and then move into rising or sitting trot, depending on which the horse feels most at ease with. After eight to ten strides the horse can be either straightened back to the track or allowed out onto a circle. As with all training care must be taken that the rider is deciding the action not the horse.

Another way to introduce shoulder in is from the spiral leg yield. As the horse spirals out and reaches the track it can be asked for a few steps of shoulder in before resuming the circle. This can be useful for horses that tend to lose impulsion into the shoulder in as it is easier to maintain the energy from the spiral. At first the angle should be kept slight, taking care to maintain the rhythm, energy and balance.

Summary

- Overall aim: for the rider to establish responsiveness, suppleness and balance in the horse.
- By developing the horse's:
  awareness of the rider's aids
  confidence in the rein so that the contact is light, elastic and consistent
  obedience to the aids in terms of forward, backward, left and right
  confidence and dexterity in its flat work.
- Method
  logical progressive schooling exercises which enable the muscles to
    remain supple and the ligaments and joints to become flexible
  carrying out the exercises in different situations to best equip the horse
    for competition

introducing the concept of direct transitions, rein back, flying change
and early lateral work.
- Lesson management
  have a clear goal
  reward achievement
  allow sufficient time to warm up and cool down.
- Likely problems
  immaturity of the horse leading to physical discomfort
  tension caused by lack of understanding
  conformation problems making exercises difficult
  rider anxiety due to lack of knowledge, physical limitations or lack of
  confidence in their ability to train the horse.

14 Lungeing and Loose Jumping

The aim of this chapter is to outline the basic skills required to work a horse both on the lunge and loose. It is a matter of personal preference how much a trainer does with a horse when it is not ridden. However, there is no doubt that being able to study the horse free of any encumbrance from the rider is fascinating and rewarding. As with any work linked to training it is essential that a clear goal is identified from the outset.

Lungeing

The horse may be lunged for a variety of reasons:

- to accustom the horse to becoming obedient to the voice and to accepting the saddle and bridle during the breaking process;
- to exercise an over-fresh horse or to exercise a horse that cannot be ridden, for example if the horse has a sore back or its regular rider is not available and it is not used to being ridden by others;
- to evaluate the horses basic paces and balance;
- to evaluate its jumping technique and attitude;
- to improve the horse either on the flat or over fences.

In order for lungeing to be beneficial the going must be good; in particular it must not be slippery. The handler and trainer must have learned how to lunge with a schoolmaster prior to undertaking the training of a young competition horse. The tack must be suitable and fit the horse. If lungeing over fences the obstacles must be suitable for the purpose.

The instructor's task is to teach the young trainer to be observant and to be able to evaluate what he or she has seen and to put it into perspective. In order to assess and evaluate the horse and then to design a training programme the young trainer must also be able to place his or her observations in an order of priority. It is often considered that lungeing is an easy option in terms of time and effort, but bearing in mind the time it takes to tack up for lungeing and that 20 minutes' actual work is probably a minimum to ensure that the horse has been properly worked, it is not an easy option at all. The horse needs to wear a bridle, lungeing cavesson and roller, boots all round and probably side reins. In addition the handler will need a lunge line and whip, should always wear gloves, and, with a strange horse or one known to be frisky, a hard hat. Suitable footwear that gives good grip and some protection should the horse tread on you is essential; trainers are not suitable.

Familiarity can breed contempt and this is probably more likely to happen with lungeing than any other area of working with horses. It is easy to become careless and people have been badly injured when lungeing so it is important not to allow the young trainer to become 'slap happy'.

Evaluating the horse's paces on the lunge

The aim is for the young trainer to be able to assess the horse's basic paces and balance initially, before moving on to assess its jump. The horse should be correctly tacked up, with solid leather side reins available but not yet fitted. The horse may be a little fresh when it first comes out, especially in strange surroundings, so it must be given time to settle down before making any decisions. This may mean that the horse canters around and has a buck or it may trot off with its tail in the air. The side reins should not be attached; the horse should simply be allowed 5 minutes or so of freedom. Once the horse has settled down it should begin to listen to the voice so that the trainer can establish a rapport with the horse and begin to assess it more systematically. When a horse is being assessed for the first time it may be useful to see all three paces demonstrated as naturally as possible, so, provided that the horse is not behaving like a hooligan, the side reins can be left off initially.

Assessment:
- The horse should have a rounded action that has scope and spring. This may be less pronounced in the event horse where roundness must not detract from speed.
- The walk should be regular, free and unconstrained with four regular hoof beats. The horse should over-track, that is the hind feet should step beyond the imprints of the fore feet.
- The trot should be regular, full of lively impulsion, elastic, naturally rhythmic and should at least track up.
- The canter should have a clear three-time beat, be rhythmic and natu-

rally well balanced. Canter is the most important gait for the jumper and experience shows that it is easier to improve a poor trot than a poor canter. Any tendency to become disunited or constantly change legs should be viewed with great suspicion or concern.

- In all three paces the horse should be in self-carriage, to a suitable degree for the stage of training. The horse should naturally carry its poll at the highest point without any tendency to hollow. The hind legs should be capable of stepping underneath the horse so that its carrying capacity can be developed reasonably easily.
- The horse should not be excessively wild or sluggish; each presents long-term training problems.
- It should accept the bit. Avoid horses that play with their tongues, with or without the side reins; this may be an incurable problem.
- The horse should travel fairly straight on the circle and look in the correct direction, with the hind feet following the front feet. If the horse carries its tail crooked the reason should be investigated promptly by a vet or back specialist.

As stated at the outset it is not easy to see everything at once and the less experienced trainer will need to develop an eye. However, as a rule of thumb, if everything looks right it probably is! If the eye is drawn to something that does not look right, then dig deeper and, above all, never be afraid to ask somebody else's opinion. Two heads are often better than one.

Once the horse has been evaluated without side reins on both the right and left reins then the side reins should be attached so that they come into contact when the horse's nose is just in front of the vertical. Check how confidently the horse accepts the contact; does it come behind the bit or resist the bit in any way? Whatever job the horse is being trained for, curing mouth problems is probably the most difficult task of all, so any major problems, such as putting the tongue over the bit, need to be addressed immediately. Less serious problems such as grinding the teeth a little or leaning on the bit and opening the mouth may not be a major defect in the jumper and can be improved with schooling.

The horse should be as straight as possible with the hind feet following the fore feet. Remember that if the untrained horse is worked on too small a circle this may be impossible for it.

Developing work on the lunge

In order to develop the horse's work on the lunge, the young trainer must be able to evaluate the horse's needs and then to prioritise them. Very often the exercises chosen may be beneficial in more than one way, so which exercise is chosen first may not be crucial.

Rhythm

Without rhythm the balance will be lost, usually because the tempo is also wrong. If the tempo is wrong the horse will not be able to utilise the impulsion effectively. Tempo is the speed of the rhythm. Some horses have such superb natural rhythm that it is almost impossible to destroy it, but the majority of horses need the trainer to find the best rhythm for them and then fit in the tempo and the impulsion.

How to find the rhythm

During the evaluation work the trainer will have observed what rhythm the horse puts itself into. In order to check that this is the horse's best rhythm the trainer can 'try out the gearbox', moving the horse up to a quicker tempo and asking him or herself: 'Does this look hurried? Is the horse falling on its forehand? Or does it now look more at ease and better able to sustain the steps?' The trainer can then slow the tempo down checking that the horse is still stepping under and not dragging its hind feet. If the pace seems laboured then the tempo is probably too slow; conversely there may be more lift to the steps and the rhythm may be more clearly pronounced. This discovery of the best rhythm is a vital tool for the trainer and the horse should be encouraged to step into its best rhythm automatically every time it works. This implies that the trainer must be absolutely sure what he or she wants.

Establishing the rhythm

Horses that find it difficult to discover a good, purposeful rhythm in trot can often be helped with the use of ground poles set on a curve with a distance of 4 ft 6 in (1.37 m) between the centre of the poles. This gives the trainer the opportunity to shorten or lengthen the steps by using a smaller or larger circle. Two sets of four poles at opposite sides of a 20 m circle are ideal, starting with the poles on the ground and then gradually raising them up to 6 in (15 cm) off the ground. Raising alternate sides can be an effective way of introducing this exercise, making sure that the poles cannot be easily dislodged. If the horse has not previously worked over poles it is advisable to start with only one pole, initially leading the horse over the pole and, as it becomes confident, stepping away a little but keeping the horse on a short rein and staying close to it. When adding more poles it is best to go from one to three as horses often try to jump two.

If Bloks or similar obstacles are available it is a good idea to introduce them now so that the horse becomes used to passing between them. It is important that the trainer is certain whether he or she is working the horse over poles to enhance the rhythm and balance or as an introduction to jumping. For the former it is recommended that the side reins are kept attached.

Developing engagement and impulsion

The most successful way to develop engagement and impulsion is to work on transitions, but this will only be effective if the horse is obedient on the lunge, especially to the voice. Start by simply asking for walk–trot–walk transitions. Initially make a transition every three circles then gradually reduce this as the horse begins to understand the exercise. Ideally the horse will have established a lively rhythmical trot, walk and then trot on again after only two or three steps of walk. The quality of the transitions is important and throughout the work the horse must always be committed forwards. The trainer must be observant and make sure that the first step is as good as the subsequent steps. If the exercise leads to a loss of rhythm it is possible that the horse is not yet ready for this work; leave it for a few weeks and then ask again. The transition to canter is particularly difficult until the horse clearly understands the commands and it may take several sessions before it realises that there is no need to rush. The acceptance of the whip by the horse is also most important. The trainer must encourage the horse to be unafraid of the whip but also to respect it. Once the transitions from pace to pace are established then transitions within the pace should be introduced, even if the stride difference seems small at first. Watch first for the reaction: does the horse clearly offer more when asked? If so the exercise will be beneficial. However, never go on for too long and ask for too many lengthened strides or the horse may fall onto its forehand and become unbalanced. Start by asking for four to six strides, building up to eight good strides.

Improving suppleness and balance

Spiralling can be introduced on the lunge in just the same way as during ridden schooling. As there is no inside leg to help, special care must be taken that the spiralling is under the trainer's control and that the small circle is not sustained for too long – two to four 10 m circles is sufficient. It is often beneficial to hold the lunge rein in two hands for this exercise as it enables the trainer to adjust the contact as the rein becomes longer or shorter depending on the size of the circle. The leading hand should always be the hand nearest the horse's nose. This exercise can be carried out in all three paces provided that the horse is sufficiently well balanced and the surface is not slippery.

The trainer should decide at the outset of the session which exercises are to be used; it is impossible and undesirable to do everything at once. The young trainer should be encouraged to study the horse and its training programme and then go from there. The halt on its own is not considered to be particularly beneficial to the jumper, but when a halt is required in order to adjust the equipment or to change the rein, then the horse should stay on the circle and wait for the trainer to go to it. This may take time to achieve and will partially depend on how well the horse has been broken.

Lungeing over fences (Figs 14.1–14.7)

Working the horse on the lunge over fences is a useful way of evaluating the horse's technique and attitude prior to being ridden over fences.

As the horse will be accustomed to working over poles, the first jump should not be too much of an event. It is often said that many roads lead to Rome; the important thing is to know where Rome is! When introducing the horse to jumping I believe nothing is wrong so long as the horse remains confident. Ideally the young trainer starts the horse over a small cross pole (1 ft 6 in, 45 cm high) with a ground pole on either side, about 1 ft 6 in (45 cm) from the cross pole. These act as groundlines and encourage the horse to make a good shape over the fence and not to get too close; they also encourage the horse to actually jump. Other trainers use a placing pole 8 ft (2.5 m) in front of the cross pole. This gives the horse a lot to think about and may confuse it initially. Bloks, jumpkins or low wings with a run-up pole are ideal to make the fence as the lunge rein will not get caught up.

The trainer must be very observant and quick on his or her feet so that the horse is not inhibited in its jump and yet remains under control. The horse should be allowed four or five straight strides when approaching the obstacle, which should ideally be placed by a wall or fence. The horse need only wear a bridle, cavesson and boots if jumping is the sole purpose of the exercise. On landing the horse should be allowed two or three straight strides before turning back onto the circle. Do not jump each time but use the circle to re-establish balance and rhythm. The horse should be worked on both reins, not forgetting to alter the run-up pole when changing the rein. This early work should be from trot, but if the horse is clearly in better

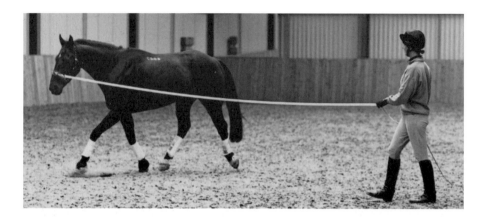

Fig. 14.1 Warming up in trot.

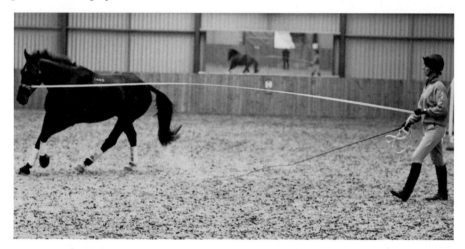

Fig. 14.2 Warming up in canter.

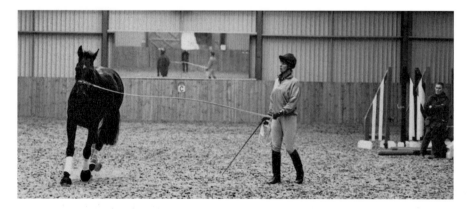

Fig. 14.3 Using spiralling to improve suppleness and balance.

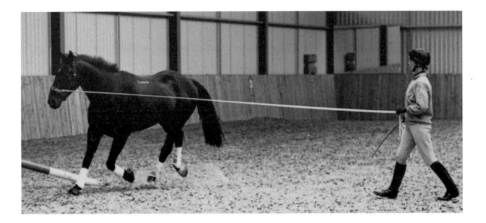

Fig. 14.4 Moving towards the fence.

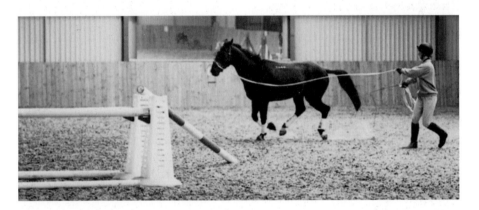

Fig. 14.5 The approach – note the need for the trainer to move with the horse.

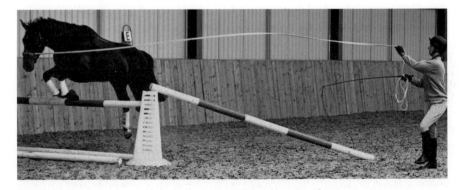

Fig. 14.6 The jump – note the movement of the trainer, allowing the horse the freedom to jump.

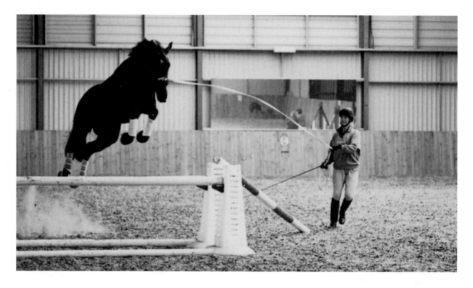

Fig. 14.7 The jump.

balance and more confident in canter it can be allowed to canter to the fence, taking care that it does not become fast and flat. In the next session the horse can progress to a vertical, building up to 2 ft 6 in (0.7 m) and keeping the groundlines. During these first sessions the trainer is mainly looking at the horse's mental attitude:

- Does the horse prick its ears and approach the fence with enthusiasm?
- If the horse knocks the fence down does it make an extra effort next time?
- Can the horse adjust its take-off platform?

Many horses do not immediately show an extravagant technique over these smaller fences; this will come later as spread fences are introduced, especially when parallels come into play. The first spread fence should ideally be a cross pole (2 ft, 60 cm in the middle) with a rail (2 ft 6 in, 0.7 m high) placed 2 ft 6 in (0.7 m) behind it, again with a groundline. The parallel can be introduced after this, building it square with groundlines either side. As long as the horse remains confident then the fences can be built up session by session, but probably the trainer should not ask the horse to jump more than twice a week. By now the trainer should have been able to assess the horse's jumping technique:

- Does the horse lower its head and neck so that the withers come up (Fig. 14.8)?
- Does the horse lift its shoulders and forearms and then fold its knees and tuck up its feet? Forelimb technique can sometimes be improved, but be wary of the horse that dangles its forearms. The lower leg usually improves with training but the forearms are more tricky.
- Does the horse 'leave its hind legs behind' and then flick them up?

If the horse does not show a good technique on the lunge check that the trainer is not inhibiting the horse in any way. If it crashes through fences with impunity it is probably not destined for the jumping world. If it refuses every time it is presented with something new it probably will not have the right attitude for the work.

Trouble shooting

If things go wrong when lungeing – the horse rushes off, turns in or whips round – then first of all ask if the trainer is at fault, for example has he or she got in front of the horse thus weakening his or her influence? Then establish that the horse is physically alright, with no signs of lameness, stiffness or other discomfort. Solving problems requires a two-pronged approach: the physical and the psychological. Mentally the trainer must always try to stay one step ahead of the horse. If the horse is strong, do not run it into the wall to stop it but gradually spiral the circle down, speaking firmly at the same time. Then thread the lunge rein from the inside bit ring over the head and attach it onto the outside bit ring. This over head check is very powerful and care must be taken not to catch the horse in the mouth when using it for jumping. If the horse turns in or whips round an assistant may be helpful to keep the horse moving forward, using another lunge whip nearer the horse. Care must be taken that the assistant does not get in a position where he or she could be kicked. An alternative is to run a second rein which runs around the outside of the horse, in effect long reining on a circle. This requires considerable skill and practice.

More advanced work

It is possible to work a horse over a bounce or double on the lunge provided that the trainer is agile and adept at the job and that the horse has a calm

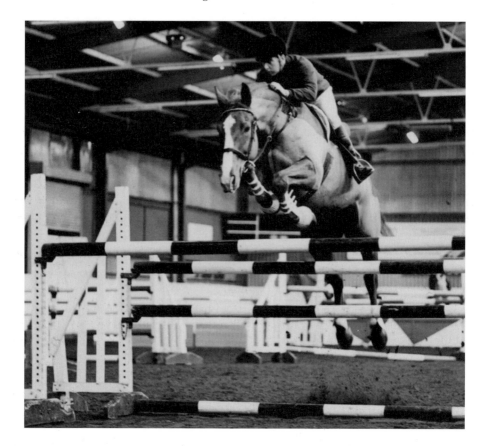

Fig. 14.8 Using the head and neck well.

attitude. However, many trainers prefer to do this loose if there are the facilities available. The dimensions of the fences should be kept small, so, for example, a vertical (2 ft 6 in, 0.7 m) to another vertical of the same height with a distance between of 18 ft (5.5 m) is ideal for the first double. Ground poles should be used. A bounce would be best at 2 ft (0.6 m) with 9 ft (2.8 m) between, using cross poles with ground poles. It may be necessary to use a placing pole at 8 ft (2.4 m) if the horse has a problem in finding a take-off zone, but normally this would be introduced when the horse is ridden.

Loose schooling

For loose schooling the trainer will need one or two assistants who are strategically placed around the arena to help the horse to stay thinking forwards and prevent it running into corners, stopping or turning round. The run up to the fence needs to be well protected to stop the horse running out at the last minute, which is dangerous for all concerned and very bad psychologically for the horse. A basic jumping lane needs to be built using jump wings and poles, high enough to discourage the horse from jumping out but not so high and gappy that it could duck underneath. The horse should wear a headcollar and boots all round and should be warmed up for at least 10 minutes prior to jumping, working evenly on both reins. If it is the sort of horse that needs to be chased for this work, it is probably not suited to it and would be better on the lunge or ridden. Others seem to enjoy it and actually have to be stopped from jumping. The trainer must be experienced and remain extremely alert to the horse and the helpers. It is easy for accidents to occur unless everyone is vigilant throughout.

Throughout the sessions, especially loose jumping, the trainer should be looking for evidence of balance and agility (Figs 14.9 and 14.10).

- Does the horse land naturally on the correct lead for the turn?
- Can the horse adjust its stride to find the best take-off platform? A horse that can only jump off a long or a short stride may be limited in top class competitions.
- Does the horse retain a natural rhythm throughout?
- Does the horse change legs fluently or just in front? If it is inclined to change behind but not in front this may indicate weakness.

The key factor, however, is that even if the horse only 'throws' one good jump a week, it is probably worth training. Very few horses make a superb job every time.

Summary

- Overall aim: for the trainer to establish confidence in the young horse and to be capable of assessing the horse both on the flat and over fences.
- By developing:
  a strategy for assessment
  good lungeing technique
  good rapport with horses and helpers
  a sound knowledge of jumping distance for young horses.
- Method
  logical progressive exercises to explore the horse's natural ability
  ensuring discipline through obedience and understanding

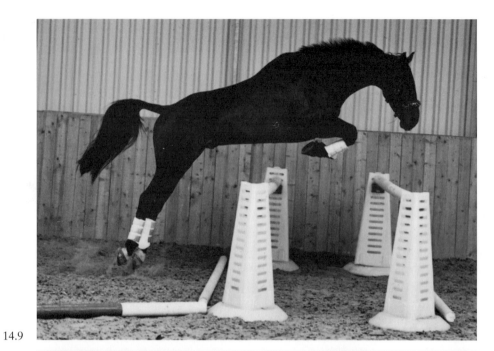

14.9

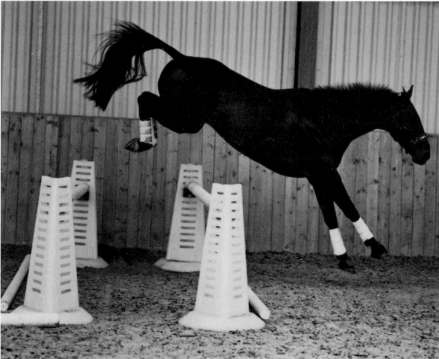

14.10

Figs 14.9 and 14.10 Evaluating the horse's technique while jumping loose.

working through exercises to enhance balance and dexterity.
- Lesson management
    clear goals with the ability to be flexible based on outcomes
    reward achievement; always stop on a good point
    keep the horse's mind calm
    allow its body to warm up and cool down
    maintain its confidence
    set out equipment beforehand
    arrange for helpers if necessary.
- Likely problems
    lack of confidence and/or ability of the horse
    lack of physical dexterity and anticipation by the trainer
    tension – physical or mental – of the horse
    lack of well-organised facilities
    poor session planning
    over-estimating the horse's ability or confidence.

15 Introducing the Young Horse to Jumping

The aim of this chapter is to explain in simple terms, step by step, how to introduce a young horse to jumping with a rider. Before jumping with a rider the horse should be capable of walk, trot and canter in balance with a fair rhythm. Ideally it should also respond to the aids which enable the rider to adjust the tempo. It is difficult to say in terms of months when this might be; all horses are going to progress at a different rate. Other factors include the experience of the trainer and whether the horse has had any mental or physical set-backs.

As explained earlier, it is not advisable for the novice rider to educate the novice horse. Ideally the rider will be balanced, supple and have jumped experienced horses up to 3 ft 7 in (1.1 m). In addition the rider should be confident and preferably the same person that has been riding the horse on the flat and has worked the horse on the lunge and loose. It is also advisable that the young horse trainer has a confirmed trainer to work with on a regular basis. It does not matter how experienced the rider is, there will always be times when a more experienced eye on the ground is invaluable.

There must be a suitable area to train the horse with good going. If the horse has to be schooled on grass this may limit how much jumping can be done in the summer. The ground is likely to be hard and may jar the young horse; if repeated too often this will affect its attitude to the work. The planning of its schooling activities needs special attention. Equally, slippery or deep going will cause problems. Few trainers have the ideal facilities, but provided that the problems are recognised and addressed then work can progress quite satisfactorily. The minimum amount of jumping equipment is probably four sets of wings, ten poles and four Bloks or equivalent. Over a period of time it is useful to buy some fillers, planks, gates, etc.

Most horses are not mature enough to start serious jump training until they are four years old, but lungeing over poles and small fences can start earlier. Ideally the young trainer should integrate the flat work and the introduction to jumping so that jumping does not become a major issue in the horse's mind. Work over trotting poles, canter poles, small fences and grids could take place two or three times a week as the purpose of these sessions is not only to educate the horse but also to strengthen it for a career that demands a great deal of developed power. The work is the same at this stage whether the horse is destined to be a show jumper or an event horse; indeed if all hunters and school horses had a similar education all riders would benefit. Certainly the better trained the horse is, the more likely it is to last for many years as both its mind and body have been progressively trained to cope with the work demanded. However, a word of warning: athletics coaches are continually reminded of the dangers of over-training the young athlete in strenuous disciplines such as gymnastics. Trainers of trainers and the trainers of horses must be equally aware of this and constantly monitor the horse's physical and mental reactions to the training programme. If the goals that have been set are too demanding then they must be adjusted; this can be difficult if sponsors or parents are placing demands on the trainer and rider.

Poles on the ground

The more subtle the introduction of the horse to the new exercise the greater the likelihood that the horse will accept it willingly and calmly. As soon as the horse can be steered safely and can walk, trot and canter in reasonable balance it can be introduced to poles on the ground. Ideally the horse will have worked over poles on the lunge. Even so the exercise should be introduced gradually, starting with single coloured poles scattered about the working area so that they can be ridden over or past. At first the horse should just be walked over the poles and any tendency to slow down on the approach should be countered by stimulating activity from the leg, backed up by the whip if necessary. A neck strap is a useful aid for the rider during all early work in case the horse makes an unbalancing bound over anything strange. The horse should be allowed to lower its head and neck on the approach, but care should be taken not to slacken the reins so much that the horse could run out or whip round. Progressing to trot, the rider should remain in a light, balanced rising trot (Fig. 15.1) and the horse should be rewarded with a pat or verbal praise when it performs well. It is vital at this stage that the young trainer is not allowed to place the horse at the poles; the horse must be trained to retain some of its own initiative at all times.

Once the horse is confident over single poles then a series can be introduced. As with the lungeing exercise build up from one pole to three, as horses are inclined to jump two poles. The poles should be placed around 4 ft 6 in (1.4 m) apart. Even though the distance is not ideal many horses benefit from being walked over the poles initially before moving on to trot. The rider should again be in a light balanced rising trot; this is easiest for the horse.

Jumping a small fence

The next move would be to introduce a small fence. Normally this would be out of trot over a cross pole with a groundline either side (Fig. 15.2). This enables the fence to be jumped from both directions.

Most young horses when faced with their first obstacle with a rider are a little uncertain and this uncertainty can manifest itself in several ways:

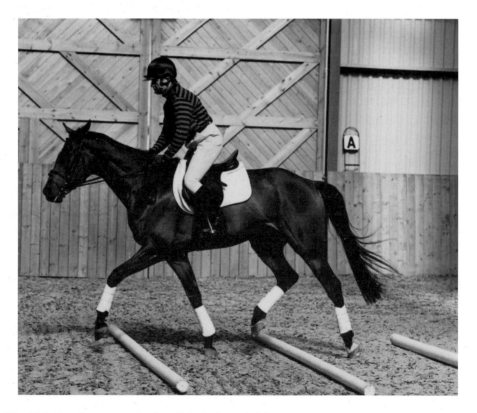

Fig. 15.1 Trotting over poles in a light balanced rising trot.

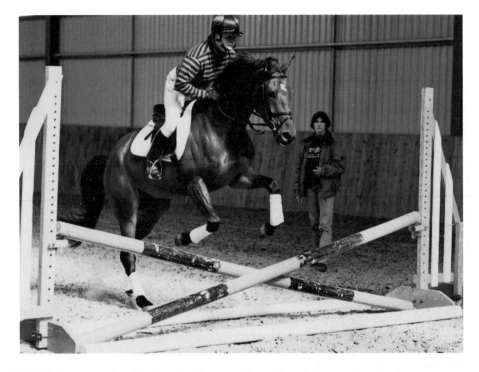

Fig. 15.2 A cross pole with a groundline on either side.

- The horse may slow down. Providing that it is still thinking forwards this may not be a problem, but often the slower the tempo the more awkward and unbalanced the jump will be.
- The horse may waver from side to side on the approach, perhaps looking to run out. The rider needs to keep enough rein contact to guide the horse in and must also ride forwards positively without losing the rhythm and balance.

Very few horses actually refuse to jump if the preparation has been thorough. If the horse does refuse, try to work out why this has happened and then take the appropriate action. For example, maybe the horse was not really looking where it was going and was taken by surprise; obviously the horse should not be chastised for this. However, if it simply refused to go forward over the fence this is disobedient and must be corrected immediately. Often, if the horse has wavered on the approach it may not jump straight and the rider must be prepared for this and try to stay as balanced as possible.

The landing can be a little unpredictable and the rider must be prepared for this also. Ideally the horse will land in canter, the rider will stay in balance and quietly go forwards to trot and come to the fence again. However, the horse may be so excited by this new experience that it lands and bucks; the rider should correct the horse but not make an issue of it. Some horses land and flop back into trot. This is not desirable as the horse should develop a positive attitude to jumping. It is therefore a good idea to delay progressing to the next stage in the horse's education until the rider can pick up canter on landing and keep the horse manoeuvrable.

Canter poles (Figs 15.3–15.5)

It is now beneficial to introduce the young horse to cantering over poles for two reasons:

(1)   to check that the canter is sufficiently well balanced to allow the horse to canter to a small fence;
(2)   a series of canter poles is an ideal way to develop the rhythm, keep the stride even and to develop the power and balance of the canter.

The trainer should take a light balanced seat in canter, keep the horse straight and to the centre of the pole, allowing the horse to find its own moment to bound over the pole. Single poles should be used in a similar manner to the way trotting poles were introduced. The exercise can then progress to three poles placed 9 ft (2.7 m) apart. After the horse has cantered over the poles two or three times on each rein the trainer should evaluate if this is the best distance for that particular horse and alter the distance if necessary. The whole purpose of the exercise is to enhance rhythm and balance and this will not be achieved if the young horse is either over-stretched or over-collected. Another eye on the ground can be invaluable here.

Raised trotting poles

The trotting pole work can be developed by raising the poles a few centimetres; raising alternate ends can be an effective way of introducing the exercise. Bloks are ideal for this work as they prevent the poles rolling, which can be alarming for the young horse. As the poles are raised the distance

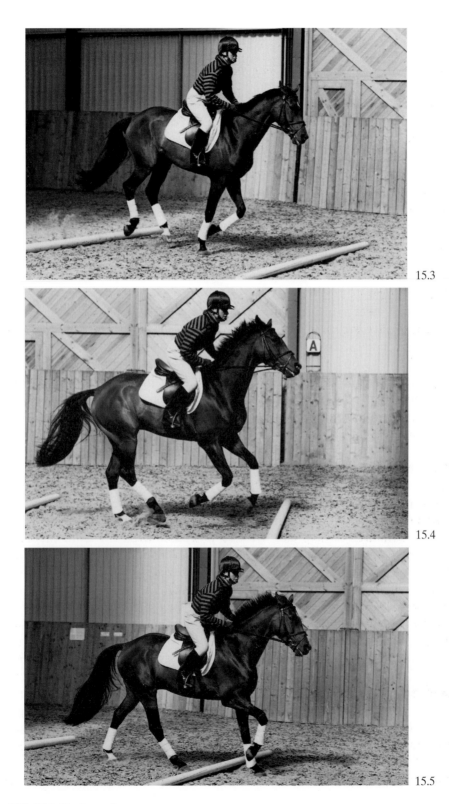

15.3

15.4

15.5

Figs 15.3–15.5 Canter poles.

between them should not be altered, creating an energetic exercise which should not be repeated too often. Ten or twelve attempts should be sufficient. Ideally, when riding over poles and small fences a light contact should be maintained throughout. If the contact is surrendered completely this can often leave the horse suddenly feeling insecure. It also requires extremely good balance from the rider to retrieve the contact softly once it has been given away.

The work can now be linked using two different exercises.

Trotting poles to a cross pole

Exercising over trotting poles to a cross pole is designed to develop the horse's agility, suppleness, balance and power. This can be done using poles on the ground or raised poles. Normally three poles are used spaced 4 ft 6 in (1.4 m) apart with a distance of 8 ft (2.4 m) from the last pole to a small cross pole. Again after two or three attempts the trainer should check that the distance between the the last trot pole and the fence suits the horse, adjusting it if necessary.

Cantering to a fence

The horse can be introduced to cantering to a fence by building a cross pole with ground lines, with the cross at about 2 ft 6 in (0.7 m) high in the centre. A small vertical can then be placed 43 ft (13 m) from the cross to allow three non-jumping strides. The vertical should have groundlines and be no more than 2 ft 6 in (0.7 m) high. The fence should be a vertical rather than a cross pole so that the horse will not have to jump higher should it veer to the side. Cross poles can be introduced once the horse is confident.

The horse has been taught to trot to a fence and land in canter, and this is exactly how the exercise using trotting poles to a cross pole should be ridden. The trainer should be aware that the horse may wander between the two fences, but providing there is enough impulsion this should not pose a problem. The trainer should try to sit as still as possible between the two fences, maintaining the contact. On landing the trainer should encourage the horse to land in canter and remain in balance.

The exercise of cantering to a fence can be developed using four or five strides of canter between the two fences. For four strides the distance used would initially be 56 ft (17 m), and for five strides it would be 67 ft

(20.4 m). Once more it is the trainer's job to evaluate how the horse is coping with these initial distances and to vary them accordingly. By using this method to introduce the horse to jumping from canter, the horse is sure where it is going to take off and everything is kept as regulated as possible.

Introducing a spread fence (Fig. 15.6)

A spread fence can be introduced in the same way and as the horse's confidence grows so the fence can be raised. Initially introduce the spread three strides from a cross pole, using a cross pole with a rail behind it as the first spread fence. This exercise should not be attempted until the horse can be kept straight and the fences should be kept small, not exceeding 2 ft 9 in (0.8 m) in height or width.

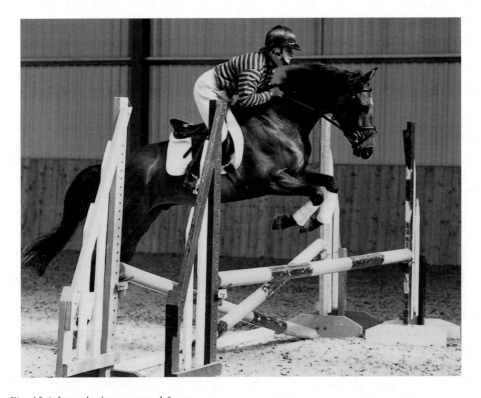

Fig. 15.6 Introducing a spread fence.

If the horse finds it difficult to regulate the strides between the fences, ground poles can be used between the fences (Figs 15.7–15.9). To get the distances right, step 9 ft (2.7 m) from the last fence towards the cross pole and add the last pole, step another 9 ft (2.7 m) and add the next pole and so on. This will ensure that the horse has enough room to land before negotiating the first pole. The first time that a horse is ridden down a line of fences including canter poles it may 'back off' as there is a lot to look at and the trainer should be ready for this and take appropriate action.

Developing athleticism

The horse's athleticism can be further developed working out of trot by introducing a 'bounce' exercise where the horse does not take a canter stride between fences, but takes off immediately on landing over the first fence. It is important that this exercise is not introduced until the horse can stay straight and is forward thinking about its jumping. The exercise can be introduced by using trotting poles to a small cross pole, then 9 ft (2.7 m) to another small cross pole. It is important that the sides of the cross are not too high as the horse may frighten itself, twisting to avoid hitting the fence. Providing that the poles are 12 ft (3.6 m) in length and the cross is no more than 2 ft 3 in (0.6 m) high in the middle, all should be well. Again the trainer should encourage the horse to land in canter and stay balanced. The number of efforts can be built up as the horse becomes stronger, but care must be taken that it does not become too fast down the grid or all the benefits will be lost.

Placing poles

There may be some horses that find it difficult to find a consistent take-off platform from trot and these horses may be helped by a placing pole in front of the fence. This should be set at around 8 ft (2.4 m) for the average horse jumping out of trot. This pole may be used later on when schooling horses that have developed minor problems, but it is important that the young horse does not learn to rely on a placing pole in order to be able to jump from trot. It is equally important that the trainer knows exactly why he or she uses any exercise and can explain the reasons to the rider.

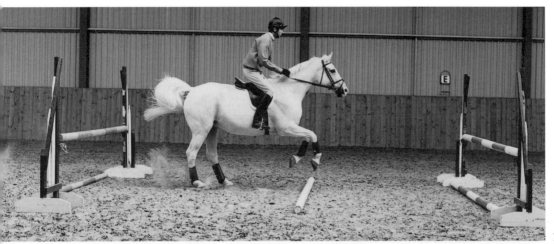

15.7

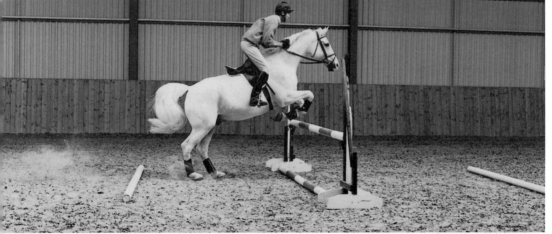

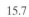

15.8

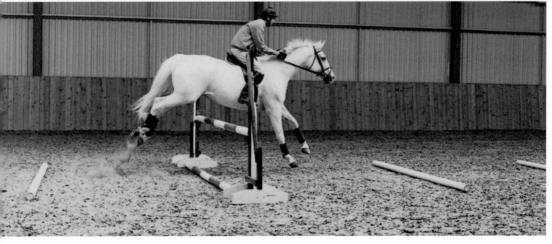

15.9

Figs 15.7–15.9 Using ground poles between fences.

Introducing fillers

The horse may now be sufficiently adept for the trainer to start to introduce fillers and other obstacles. However, it is important that the horse can jump confidently and in good style before it is asked to tackle a potentially difficult situation. Ideally the first few fillers would be rustic – perhaps small brush fences or hurdles. They should be no bigger than 2 ft 9 in (0.8 m) so that the horse will still be able to jump them even if it has had a major 'spook' at them.

The first few times the fillers are used it is often easier for the horse if they are placed either side of the fence so that the horse jumps between them. They can be gradually closed up so that the horse has to jump over them. This may not be necessary with every new filler, but is a wise precaution when introducing the concept or meeting particularly 'spooky' fillers such as sharks' teeth. Although work has been done on the horse's eyesight, there is still much that is not known. It is believed that although horses cannot distinguish colour as we would understand it, they are very sensitive to contrasts. It is reasonable to assume that just as humans vary in their perception of colour, contrast and shape, so do individual horses.

Doubles and combinations

Doubles and combinations should be introduced as just another schooling exercise with the fences kept low and inviting and distances that are comfortable for the individual horse. There is some debate over which the horse finds easier: a one stride or two stride distance. A two stride distance gives both the horse and the trainer more time to adjust. The exercise should be introduced in the same way using the same format as for the three stride distance in canter. The horse now knows that it lands in canter, stays straight and looks for the next fence. Initially an ideal distance for two non-jumping strides is 33 ft (10 m) and for one non-jumping stride is 21 ft (6.4 m). Again these distances are guidelines. By now the trainer should know if the horse is long, short or average striding, and adjustments can be made at the outset. The key is to build up the horse's confidence so that it makes the correct number of strides.

Cantering over fences

When the horse is introduced to cantering over small fences it is important that the fences are simple with clearly defined groundlines. The trainer should establish the best possible canter, with a good rhythm and try to keep this all the way to the fence. He or she should not try to influence the take-off point, allowing the fence to come naturally to the horse. The horse does not need to take off at exactly the same point every time; a small variation is quite acceptable. The most important job of the trainer is to maintain the rhythm and balance. As the horse's training progresses the trainer can begin to ask the horse to jump the fence from a gentle curve, onto a gentle curve, always aiming to stay in the centre of the fence. Jumps can be gradually linked together, carefully monitoring the horse's reaction and quickly seeking solutions to any problems that might arise.

Even at this early stage the horse should be encouraged to land on the correct lead; usually the rider looking in the correct direction and opening the rein will be sufficient. If the horse finds this difficult to understand then working on a curve is often the best way forward. Every effort must be made not to let the horse approach the fence disunited.

The horse should now be able to link together eight to ten fences, including a double, without losing its rhythm, balance and concentration. When it can do this and has jumped some fillers it is ready to take to another schooling venue or a clear round jumping competition. Try to avoid shows that have small jumping rings, flimsy fences or badly built courses. A horse's first experience at a show needs to be positive so that the trainer can continue to develop the horse's technique and further build its confidence.

Cross-country fences (Figs 15.10–15.12)

Introducing cross-country fences to the young horse can be done in various ways depending on the opportunities that are available. It is often very comforting to the young horse to have a schoolmaster, especially when first hacking out. If the facilities are there this is the ideal time to introduce the horse to jumping small logs, easy ditches and walking through streams or fords. The ditches must be clearly defined and not more than 2 ft 6 in (0.7 m) across, so that even if the horse is very hesitant it can be encouraged to jump from a standstill if necessary. The way in which the potential event horse tackles its first ditch will tell you much about its boldness. The best horses are usually very calm and matter-of-fact about everything and rarely refuse at a new type of obstacle. Whether tackling ditches or crossing water with the inexperienced horses, avoid boggy ground as this is frightening for them.

When the horse can canter to single obstacles with confidence, schooling over small cross-country jumps can begin. The order in which the novice

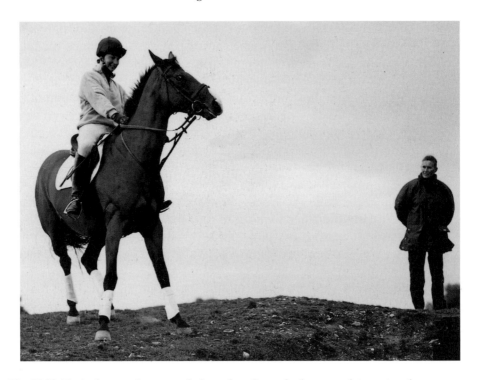

Fig. 15.10 Typical young horse confusion when first asked to negotiate a step down.

rider was introduced to riding cross-country does equally well for the young horse. The ability to maintain balance and the gradual build-up of confidence is just as important for both horse and rider.

In Switzerland one of the largest training centres introduce their young horses to cross-country fences in hand, often as young as three years old. The fences are specially designed so that the trainer can go past and lead the horse over, or in the case of ditches the trainer steps over and the horse follows. Each horse is allocated a young trainer and is led on a rein about 10 ft (3 m) long, which is threaded from the right bit ring, under the chin and through the left bit ring. There is also an extra helper with a bucketful of titbits. With an experienced horse leading the cavalcade, the horses and trainer follow the lead file, walking over logs, hedges and ditches, none of which exceed 2 ft 6 in (0.7 m). The trainer goes first, pays out the rein and the horse follows. The horse has built up so much trust in its trainer that it is prepared to follow him or her virtually anywhere. The horses are rewarded frequently and seem to really enjoy the work, treating it as a 'jolly' rather than coercion. The horses also tackle quite large banks with-

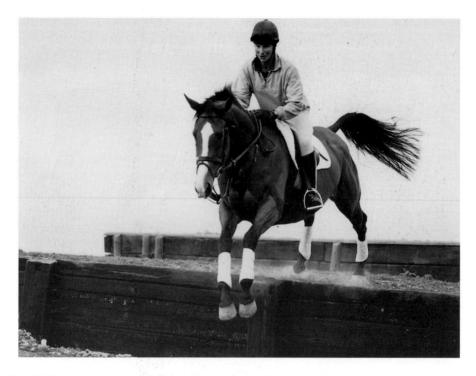

Fig. 15.11 Once the horse understands, she jumps down confidently.

out rushing off the top, being quite happy to wait until their trainer asks them to follow them off the bank. The horses may start these sessions as soon as six weeks after being broken in. Of course, the trainer has to be fit as they often trot of the horse between the obstacles! However, these horses come to jumping with riders, both-cross country and in the stadium, with utmost confidence.

Summary

- Overall aim: to educate the novice horse to a point where it is ready for its first clear round competition.
- By:
    providing a progressive, reasoned training structure with clear guide-
        lines of how to progress from ground poles to single fences
    introducing canter through related distances
    starting the horse over fillers, doubles and cross-country fences.

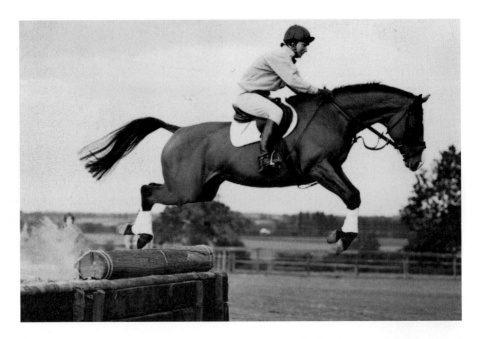

Fig. 15.12 A green horse making an exaggerated jump off a bank – note the rider allowing freedom of the head and neck.

- · Method
  concentration on the principles of rhythm, balance and confidence
  developing a sound, correct technique from the horse.
- · Lesson management
  clear goals – developing the trainer's ability to evaluate when to progress and when to amend the exercise or the training programme
  emphasis on building confidence and rewarding achievement
  making the most of facilities and opportunities.
- · Likely problems
  lack of facilities
  loss of confidence of horse or trainer
  physical problems with the horse
  over-ambitious training programme, perhaps caused by external pressures.

16   Developing Athletic Jumping

The aim of this chapter is to explain in detail the role of athletic jumping in the schooling of horse and rider for jumping. Athletic or gymnastic jumping is a vital part of the training of all jumping horses. However, in order to be a truly effective aid to development it needs to be specifically linked to the individual partnership.

Only by studying the performance of the horse and rider combination can the trainer decide which is the right exercise to concentrate on.

There are a wide range of athletic jumping exercises:

- Related distances of three to six strides.
- Doubles and combinations of one or two strides.
- Curved and straight grids, including bounces.
- Ground poles.
- A-frames, descending parallels, etc.
- Rider exercises.

Many of these remedial exercises may not appear to have immediate benefit; several weeks of schooling should be undertaken before abandoning hope. The exercises can be suited to the amount of equipment available, but a minimum would probably be three sets of wings and ten poles. Even with this there would be a great deal of shifting of equipment and the exercises for each training session would have to be carefully planned in advance. While having thought out a lesson beforehand is good teaching practice it is not always possible, for example, if the trainer is taking a clinic and having to evaluate unknown horses and riders and plan the best programme for them on the spot. Bloks are excellent for ground poles and placing fences as they keep the poles secure. Poles should not be either too light or too heavy; the former encourage the horse to be careless, while the latter can hurt the horse if it makes a mistake. A diameter of 3–4 in (7–10 cm) is ideal. If possible poles should be both rustic and painted. A couple of planks are also useful as this is a fence that horses can be careless about when in the ring.

Most of the work done over fences must be readily transferable to the competition environment. Thus the large proportion of the work should be done in canter unless a specific problem is being addressed, such as the horse having a very 'hot' temperament.

The equine athlete, just like its human counterpart, needs to keep its body supple and fit. Human athletes do not always know what is best for their own bodies and rely on their coaches for guidance. It is easy to appreciate that those working with horses encounter complex problems and only have their own skills to try to identify the needs of the horse. Riders may not always know what is most beneficial for themselves or their horses, adding further complications for the trainer.

The trainer needs to take care in his or her approach to developing athleticism; the grid is not the panacea for all problems. However, most horses do benefit from some form of athletic training, especially during their formative years. This method of schooling is also useful if problems arise. The days of rapping and jumping barbed wire poles are, or should be, long gone. Event horses also benefit from regular athletic work; they have to gallop and tend to get onto the forehand. Regular remedial work will help get back their 'shape' over a fence and keep their reactions quick.

Modern show jumping courses tend to be complex in their distances and are built with light poles in shallow cups. This was particularly well illustrated at the 1996 Olympic Games in Atlanta. The course, built by Linda Allen of the USA, was widely acclaimed as brilliant because the demands made tended to be more technical, rather than simply jumping huge unforgiving fences. Horses need to be adjustable and supple in order to perform at world level.

It cannot be over-emphasised how important it is that trainers are able to measure and interpret the distances between fences accurately. Trainers must regularly check their own stride against a tape measure to ensure accuracy. They must also be familiar with the distances used by course builders in different situations; they should take the opportunity to walk a course and then ask the course designer to confirm their interpretations. Course builders are often delighted to have someone to help them build the course before a competition and this sort of opportunity should be taken whenever possible. Trainers should discuss with riders the problems that have been set and how their horses coped. Watching televised show jumping and taking note of the heights and distances will help trainers add to their knowledge and understanding of show jumping.

Surfaces

The surface that is being worked on may enhance a horse's performance or possibly detract from it. Given a choice the trainer should always opt for the best: old turf or a well maintained, even artificial surface. Lack of rain may make grass very hard or sand very deep and the nature of the exercises set must take this into account and be adjusted as necessary.

Choosing the exercise

The rushing horse
As with all problem solving, the trainer must first try to pinpoint the cause of the problem. Initially he or she should watch and assess the rider and horse working on the flat and then over two or three fences. The trainer should question the rider to check whether this is a well established problem or one that has developed as the horse progressed. The trainer should also observe the horse and rider to establish the following:

- Are there any physical problems with the horse?
- Does the horse look level?
- Does it look very tight in its back?
- Does it look keen and enthusiastic or anxious and sharp?
- Does it accept the bridle happily?
- Is the rider at ease or is he or she nervous or afraid? This can happen if the rider has been over-faced, especially as a child.

To try to steady the rushing horse is perhaps the most common problem that the trainer is asked to resolve. Assuming that the rider is competent to do more or less what the trainer asks, the trainer should explain at the outset that the problem will not be solved in one session. It will take many weeks of patience and consistency of approach before the horse will reliably stop rushing the fences.

Most horses do pay more attention and therefore slow down if poles on the ground are used as part of the exercise. The eventual height of the fences will depend on the experience of the partnership, but the fences must always start low. A good introductory fence is a small cross pole (2ft6in, 0.7m in the middle) placed 8ft (2.4m) from a ground pole. The rider should approach in trot and if the horse rushes at the fence he or she should turn the horse away. This should be continued, patiently circling away, right and left, until the horse is fairly calm and will remain in trot on the approach to the fence. Once the horse has jumped the fence it is most important not to pull the horse up sharply on landing, but that a calm rhythmic trot is established as soon as possible. The horse should be worked off both reins and the fence raised according to the horse's attitude. However, progress should be made fairly quickly. Probably after four jumps the nature of the exercise should be subtly changed, as many horses get more and more excited if the exercise stays the same.

A pole placed on the landing side of the fence is often a useful way to steady the first landing stride and to promote a bascule over the fence. This pole should be approximately 12 ft (3.6 m) away from the fence. As the horse progresses a square oxer can be introduced at around 3 ft 3 in (1 m) high. This can be gradually opened out to promote both stretch and bascule together. These exercises would be suitable for an improvement programme for a horse competing in British Novice or Pre-novice Horse Trials. The heights and spreads can be adjusted as necessary. If the horse has the habit of taking off in front of the placing pole and the rider is unable to prevent this without being rough, then a pole at 18 ft (5.5 m) can be introduced (Fig. 16.1). This will allow the horse a canter stride between the fence and the pole. This exercise can be used to help regulate the horse to the fence once canter commences. The rider should just maintain the canter rhythm and meet the pole out of the stride quite naturally. The contact should be lightly maintained throughout, only releasing sufficient rein to allow the horse to jump without inhibition. All exercises should be carried out smoothly with no excessively strong aids at any time. Certainly corrective transitions, including rein back, can and should be used, but calmly and systematically.

The keen horse can now progress to a three-stride distance to check if the rider can maintain the rhythm evenly between the two fences (Fig. 16.2). Table 16.1 shows the jumping distances suitable for most horses. A square oxer about 3 ft 3 in (1 m) high can be built 45 ft (13.7 m) after the fence used in the previous exercise (Fig. 16.1). The approach should be in canter and the trainer can ask the rider to be aware of the rhythm and to count the strides between the two fences. Depending on the experience of the rider this may be done out loud or under the breath.

If the horse is still too keen between the two fences and the rider cannot steady it by just bringing the shoulders up and feeling down the rein, then two poles can be added on the ground to regulate the stride. The distance between the poles is normally based on a 12 ft (3.6 m) stride, allowing 9 ft (2.7 m) in front of the second fence for the take-off. As with all exercises the

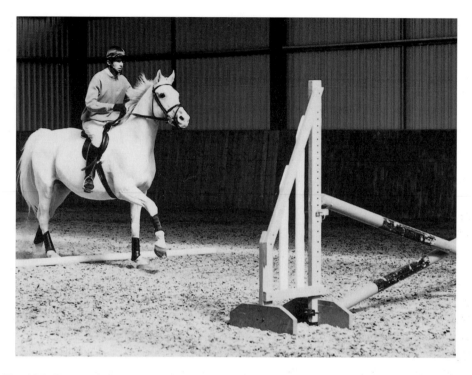

Fig. 16.1 Canter placing pole.

Table 16.1 Jumping distances suitable for most horses.

	Feet	Metres	Yards
Placing pole to a fence (trot and canter)			
bounce	8	2.5	
1 canter stride	18	5.5	
Between fences (trot or canter)			
bounce	12	3.7	4
1 stride	21	6.4	7
2 strides	33	10.1	11
3 strides	45	13.7	15
4 strides	57	17.4	19
Pole on the landing side after a fence	12	3.7	4
Canter poles	9	2.7	3
One non-jumping stride	12	3.7	4

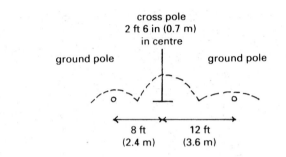

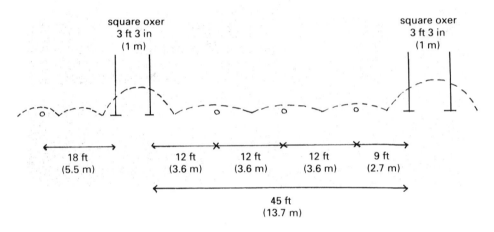

Fig. 16.2 An exercise for a rushing horse.

trainer needs to study the horse's reaction and amend the exercise as necessary for it to be of maximum benefit to the horse.

If the rider has initiated this tendency for the horse to rush by 'firing' the horse at the fence then it is valuable to go back to basics and ask the rider to count the rhythm well before the fence. The rider should count at least six strides before the fence, but up to twenty is valuable. The rider should count from one upwards and resume counting on landing. It is remarkable how many riders are not actually synchronised with their horses, but either in front or behind them. The riders who fire their horses tend to be in front of the rhythm.

Another exercise which should only be practised with confident and experienced riders is for the trainer to position him or herself about three strides from the fence and ask the riders to look at him or her as they pass (Fig. 16.3). This takes their eye off the fence and they will realise that the horse does not need violent urging in the last three strides. It works equally well if

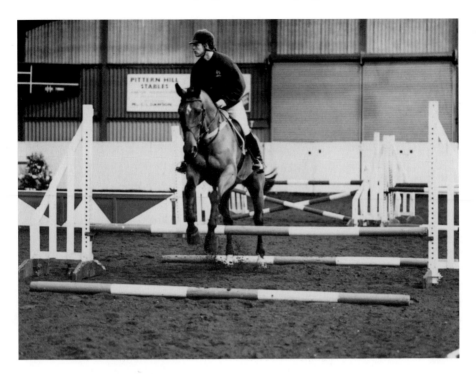

Fig. 16.3 Looking at the trainer.

the rider is asked to look up and ahead, over the normal eyeline, perhaps to another fence at least 4 ft (1.2 m) high. The horse should not need to be fixed on a 'spot' to jump from and will perform much more consistently if the rhythm is highlighted.

The rushing horse should be schooled as much as possible around fences at home, not jumping every time, but trying to make the situation of jumping as unexciting as possible. At a show these horses are often best if only given a few practice fences so that they do not become too excited.

The horse that tends to flatten or hollow

Flattening and hollowing often go hand in hand with rushing so the exercises used to help can often be similar to those already outlined. However, trainers who are involved in schooling horse and rider for horse trials should remember that excessive basculing is not really desirable when going cross-country; it is both time-consuming and rather nerve-racking at drops into water! As before the trainer must try to identify why the horse is hollow and ask whether it affects the horse's efficiency. For most horses being hollow does limit their technique and effectiveness over a fence, but just occasionally a horse will jump less successfully if its style is changed by the rider or trainer. Similarly there are human athletes that have a slightly unorthodox style and yet are world class.

The bounce (Fig. 16.4)
The exercises already mentioned will help improve the horse's bascule, but the bounce can also be used. However, the bounce should be introduced with care, initially using 12 ft (3.6 m) between the two elements. Experience has also shown it best to have a cross pole to a vertical until the horse is quite clear about what it is doing. The jumps should start low, the cross being 2 ft 6 in (0.7 m) in the middle and the vertical being 3 ft (0.9 m) high. The exercise should begin in trot using a placing pole 8 ft (2.4 m) in front of the cross pole. The exercise can be repeated in canter once horse and rider are confident. If the 8 ft (2.4 m) placing pole is being used in canter, the trainer must ensure that the horse and rider can do this at a single fence before taking on the bounce. The trainer must check that the rider is not inhibiting the horse's attempt to bascule in any way. A maximum of three bounces is probably sufficient and personal preference is to only use verticals or cross poles, preferring to leave spreads for a one or two stride situation. Two or three bounces can form a satisfactory start to a grid which can then comprise low, wide oxers to encourage the horse to round over the fence. An example is shown in Fig. 16.4. Start with the oxers 3 ft 3 in (1 m) square and then adjust according to the horse's response.

If the rider is inclined to inhibit the horse and not give the rein sufficiently then it is often beneficial to ask the rider to knot the reins and put them on the horse's neck as they approach the placing pole. The hands should then move in the normal following position and the reins should be picked up on landing over the last fence. Most horses do not run out, and providing that

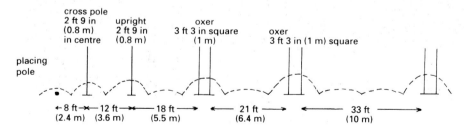

Fig. 16.4 Improving bascule: a grid incorporating a bounce exercise.

the reins are accessible the rider can retrieve them if necessary. Of course, the trainer must have judged that the horse and rider are sufficiently competent before attempting this sort of exercise.

Vertical to oxer

Another exercise that can be useful for the horse that hollows is to build a small vertical at around 3 ft 3 in–3 ft 6 in (1–1.05 m) and then an oxer 18 ft (5.5 m) away. The oxer is built with the front rail higher than the back (Fig. 16.5), starting with the front rail at about 3 ft 6 in (1.05 m) and the back rail at 3 ft (0.9 m) with a spread of 3 ft 6 in (1.05 m). The front rail should also have a dropper pole. The exercise can be increased in difficulty by

*   shortening the distance;
*   widening the oxer;
*   raising the front rail of the oxer.

This exercise is also valuable for improving the hind leg technique, if the horse pulls through too quickly or is flat.

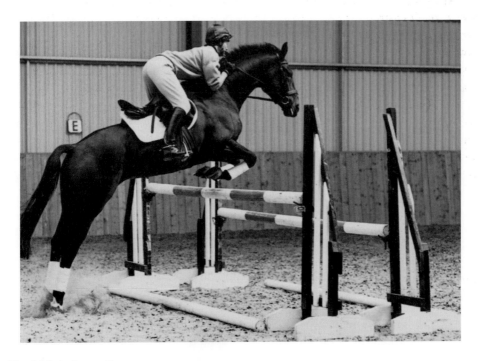

Fig. 16.5 A descending oxer.

The horse that does not snap up its front legs on take-off or use the shoulders sufficiently

This problem is often closely linked to the problem of hollowing. Some horses never learn to use their forearms as classically as one would like, while others are just a little idle or casual in their approach. The latter can sometimes be startled into action; the descending oxer can help here. Another useful exercise is the A-frame which consists of taking two poles and resting them on the supported jump pole to make an 'A' shape (Fig. 16.6). The exercise should begin with the ends well apart, gradually closing the top of the 'A'. There should be a drop pole to fill in the bottom of the fence. The A-frame is often most effective when used as part of a double or related distance. The trainer must advise the rider that this exercise often makes the horse 'back off' substantially, so a firm leg is needed to back up the rhythm and to ensure that the tempo is maintained.

Under no circumstances should the rider be allowed to pull the horse off the ground with the reins. The horse must learn to take care of itself and if it is consistently careless or jumps in a dangerous manner, it is best to admit that jumping is not its forte. Some trainers recommend placing a pole diago-

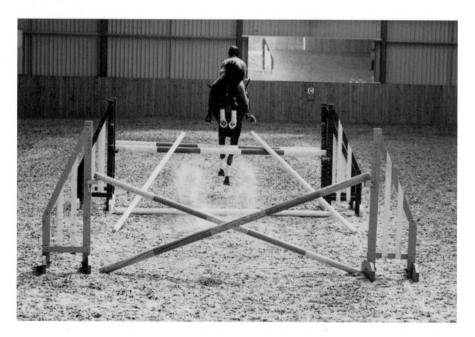

Fig. 16.6 A young horse jumping her first A frame – note the effect!

nally across the top of a wide parallel, but it must be remembered that this pole could get caught in the horse's legs, causing an accident, and this exercise is not recommended for use by developing trainers.

The horse that lacks confidence and does not go forwards

Most of the exercises outlined up till now are designed to teach the horse to shorten and become more agile. There are times, however, when horses lack confidence and are short striding, thus finding it difficult to put in the correct strides between doubles, combinations and related distances. These horses are best improved out in the open to encourage them to open the stride. The trainer will need to work on a number of aspects to develop the horse's ability to lengthen the stride and use its scope efficiently. Once more the trainer must check the rider's technique to make sure that the rider is not encouraging the horse to be inhibited or condoning the practice of putting in an extra stride.

These horses often need to work in a stronger tempo and develop their responsiveness to the rider's aids, especially the forward driving aids. Surprisingly, sitting in the saddle and driving does not always increase acceleration, so the best way to promote responsiveness needs to be identified by trial and error. Small fences that encourage forward, flowing jumping are best, for example ascending oxers. The spread can be gradually increased from 3 ft 3 in (1 m) until the horse is making an effort but does not look either afraid or uncertain. For a very short striding horse a three stride distance of 43 ft (13 m) would be used, with an ascending oxer going in at around 3 ft 3 in–3 ft 6 in (1–1.05 m) high and a vertical going out with a groundline 3 ft 3 in (1 m) in front of the fence. The horse should be kept moving up to the oxer in a strong tempo but still rhythmic, balanced and 'in front of the leg'. On landing this free flowing movement should be maintained so that the horse gets to the second fence easily. The distance between the two fences can be gradually increased at each session until the horse can cope with 48 ft (14.6 m). The same principle can be applied to the two stride double, starting with a distance of 30 ft (9.1 m) and gradually increasing the distance to 36 ft (11 m). For a one stride double start with a distance of 21 ft (6.4 m) and increase it to 25 ft (7.6 m).

The whole philosophy here must be to build up confidence, so the trainer must encourage the rider to take time and not to progress to affiliated competition until he or she is confident that the horse can jump the course as set by the course designer. Some of these horses will benefit from cross-country training, if they are sufficiently confident. This encourages them to think forward and ahead.

To develop straightness, agility and manoeuvrability

The ideal competition horse should be happy to be directed by its rider to go and jump a fence at a particular spot. The following exercises can be used for all levels of riders. The level of horse and rider competence determines the size and complexity of the fences.

Exercise 1

The first exercise utilises a 30 m circle; if working in a school that is 66 ft (20 m) wide an oval shape should be used. A fence is placed at two opposite points of the circle (Fig. 16.7). The rider chooses which part of the fence is to be jumped and then works on the circle accordingly. This exercise is very helpful in improving rhythm as the horse should take the same number of strides on each attempt if the same line is taken. This exercise can also be used to introduce increasing and decreasing the stride length. This should not be attempted until the rider is confident of maintaining a regular rhythm of his or her choice.

Exercise 2

The second exercise uses single fences (Fig. 16.8), with the trainer or rider determining where to go after jumping the first fence. The exercise works best on a distance of three strides (45 ft, 13.7 m). The exercise would start using simple verticals, the height depending on the experience of the horse and rider, but probably 3 ft 6 in–3 ft 9 in (1.05–1.1 m). These can then be expanded to include gates, planks and oxers. The trainer should let the rider experiment coming straight to the first fence and then turning, or angling the first fence, ideally working in canter. If the fences are first set up so that the

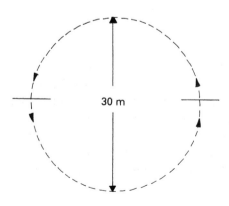

Fig. 16.7 Circle exercise: developing straightness and manoeuvrability.

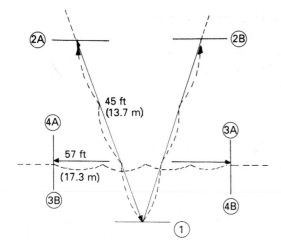

Fig. 16.8 Single fences exercise: developing straightness and manoeuvrability.

distance of 45 ft (13.7 m) is taken from the mid-point of the first fence to the mid-point of the second fence, then the rider can vary the route slightly to allow more distance between the two fences, if the horse needs it. This exercise can be further developed by turning back or across to another fence. Ideally this third fence should be able to be linked together; depending on the width of the fences the distance could be three strides (45 ft, 13.7 m) or four strides (57 ft, 17.3 m).

To improve accuracy
Improving accuracy is useful for both cross-country jumping and jump-offs. Small exercises can be built in the school or field. In order to jump accurately the trainer must teach the horse and rider combination to trust each other, so that when the horse is put on a line it will stay there.

Arrowheads
A useful exercise for improving accuracy is to build a narrow fence (Figs 16.9 and 16.10), initially using poles and wings to direct the horse to the fence. Bloks are ideal for this as they are quite safe if the horse veers off-line. The novice horse or rider should be introduced to the exercise using the guiding poles; as confidence increases the arms can be widened and finally removed. The more advanced horse and rider can then jump the fence from the other direction, with the arms going away. This simulates the arrowhead situation cross-country.

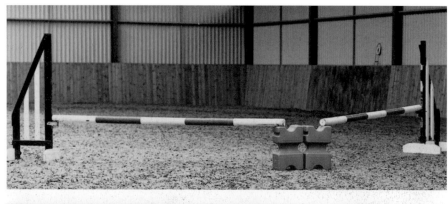

16.9

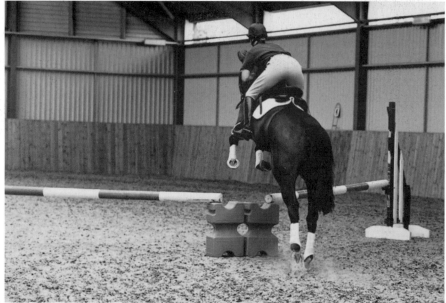

16.10

Figs 16.9 and 16.10 Arrowhead.

Corners

Corners can be built using Bloks for the corner and wings or stands for the extremities (Fig. 16.11). A drop pole can be added to give riders greater confidence of the take-off point. The trainer should start with the angle closed and only when the pupil is consistently approaching on the same line should the angle be opened up. These fences should be kept small as the principle is the key factor rather than the height and width.

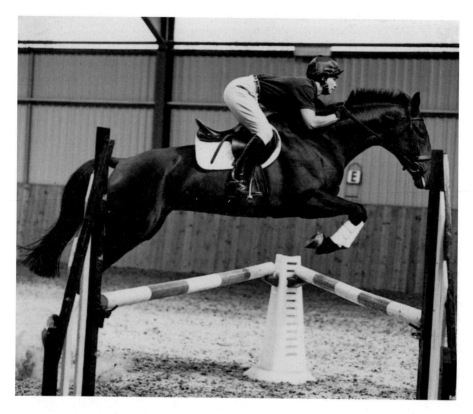

Fig. 16.11 Corner.

Jumping at an angle (Fig. 16.12)

Jumping at an angle is necessary both for cross-country and for riding the jump-off in show jumping competitions. It must be remembered that jumping across fences can lead to one of the horse's legs being lower than the other. This applies equally to forelimbs and hindlimbs. Jumping across parallels increases the width, so the ability of both rider and trainer to estimate the horse's ability is vital. As with all exercises jumping at an angle should be introduced gently, just taking an oblique line from five or six strides out, and landing securely before turning. Gradually increase the oblique line until the horse and rider are stretched in terms of accuracy and consistency. Separately introduce shorter turns onto an oblique line and turning on landing. Quite clearly these exercises should not be attempted until the horse is sufficiently balanced to make flying changes on the turns.

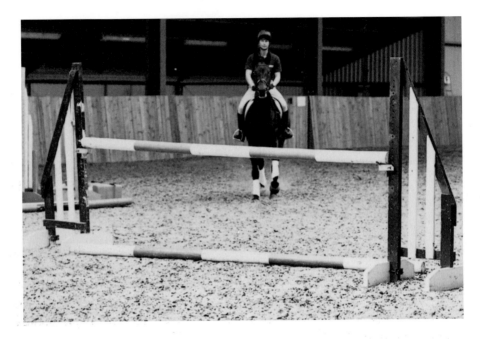

Fig. 16.12 Angled fence.

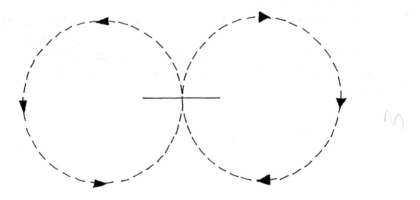

Fig. 16.13 Double circle.

Circles (Fig. 16.13)

The rider approaches a vertical fence on a circle and either stays on the circle or changes the rein to pick up another circle. The height of the fence will depend on the competence of the horse and rider and the size of the circle will be commensurate with the horse's balance, but should be a minimum of

66 ft (20 m). The exercise can be carried out in trot or canter according to the level of training.

Serpentine (Fig. 16.14)
The exercise involves cantering or trotting a serpentine over three verticals set in a straight line 39–49 ft (12–15 m) apart, centre line to centre line.

Figure-of-eight (Fig. 16.15)
The horse and rider jump two verticals set opposite each other, describing a figure-of-eight and making a total of three jumping efforts. The jumps should be set approximately 49 ft (15 m) apart, centre to centre.

Zig-zag (Fig. 16.16)
This exercise consists of three or four vertical jumps built at right-angles to each other to form a zig-zag pattern. The rider starts on either the left or right rein in canter at one end of the zig-zag and jumps each vertical straight across the centre, landing on the correct leg, jumping each element once. All the loops between the fences should be the same size. This is particularly useful for jump-off practice.

The Mercedes (Fig. 16.17)
This exercise would normally be carried out in canter but can be a good exercise from trot for novice riders to improve their presentational skills. The exercise involves three verticals set at an angle of 120° to each other. The rider may start on either rein over any of the verticals, jumping each element once.

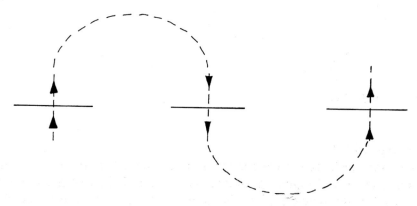

Fig. 16.14 Serpentine.

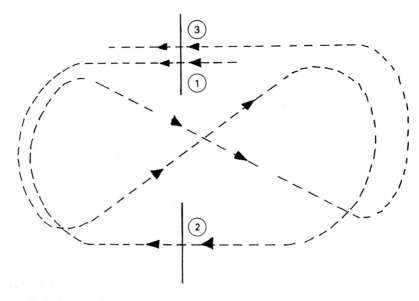

Fig. 16.15 Figure-of-eight.

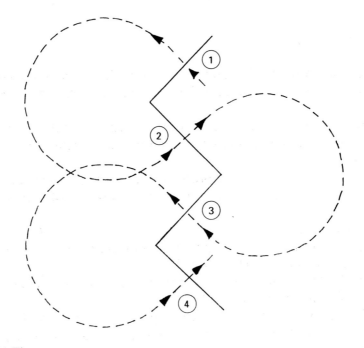

Fig. 16.16 Zig-zag.

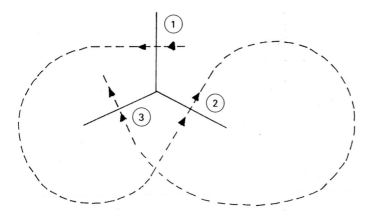

Fig. 16.17 Mercedes.

For novice riders these last five exercises could be scaled down, but the hallmarks of accuracy, rhythm and consistency should not be lost. All these exercises should emphasise rhythm, approach and the balance of horse and rider.

Summary

- Overall aim: to enable the trainer to choose suitable exercises to develop the horse and rider in order for them to reach their maximum potential.
- By:
    providing structured, reasoned exercises that are relevant to almost any problem that might be encountered when jumping.
- Method
    evaluation of the individual problem and tackling this in a way suitable for the temperament, experience and confidence of both horse and rider.
- Lesson management
    ensuring a suitable venue with sufficient facilities is available
    planning ahead as much as possible
    being decisive with regard to heights and distances so that any helpers are directed clearly but politely
    taking decisions as to how far to progress – never go too far
    checking that the rider is always in full agreement at each stage of the lesson.

- Likely problems
  lack of facilities
  underestimating the problem
  over-estimating the horse and/or rider's experience
  over-ambitious exercises and not stopping early enough
  physical problems for horse or rider
  failing to establish the rider's confidence in the trainer.

17 Competition Riding

The aim of this chapter is to focus on the needs of the competitor. These needs start long before he or she gets to the actual show or event. During training the trainer will have got to know the pupil and how he or she is likely to react at competitions. The trainer will probably have been involved in the planning of the competition season and in the setting of both long- and short-term goals. When the programme has to be altered, perhaps due to training setbacks or the cancellation of a show, the competitor will need the trainer to help with the rescheduling. The trainer also may have to help maintain the rider's motivation. Young riders, especially children, tend to get very anxious before important competitions. Riders need to be encouraged to look after themselves in terms of their physical needs; they must eat properly and sleep adequately. Often children find it difficult to accept this sort of discipline from their parents; however, it may be acceptable from their trainer, particularly if the trainer has been a competition rider him or herself. Having the will to win is vital. Having the will to prepare is also essential and the two cannot be divorced.

Handling stress

Competition involves stress. The best way to handle that stress is to be prepared both mentally and physically. This is true whether it is a novice rider at their first show or an international competitor and similar principles apply. Potential problems should be worked out at home before going to the competition. Here the trainer can help by going through the 'what if' scenarios so that the rider is prepared in advance with a positive plan of action.

The trainer's role

The trainer's role at a competition is to:

- ensure the rider arrives prepared;
- help the rider overcome nerves;
- walk the course;
- motivate the rider;
- protect the rider from outside influences;
- help the rider warm up;
- be there afterwards, win or lose.

Walking the course

Many newcomers to competition worry about forgetting the course. The trainer can help overcome this fear by getting the rider to memorise the course and then talk it through with the trainer. The rider should be able to recite the course from beginning to end, select any fence and remember which fence comes before and after it.

Another vital factor for both the show jumping and cross-country phases is time. The trainer can advise where time can be saved by taking an economical track to a fence, or where on the cross-country course it would be safe to gallop on and make up time. Alternatively the trainer could also point out where it would be important not to take chances because of the nature of the going, terrain or complexity of the fence.

Cross-country

Walking the course correctly is essential for a good ride cross-country. The aim is for the rider to:

- familiarise him or herself with the route;
- look at the fences;
- decide the approach to the fence;
- decide the pace and speed of the approach;
- decide how and where to jump the fences;
- walk the alternatives;
- look at the way in which the fences influence each other;
- determine the length of the course;
- assess the terrain;
- assess the going;
- assess other factors such as the position of the sun and natural hazards;

- determine the position of the start and finish.

At a three-day event there is normally an official course walk the day before the competition starts. Competitors are driven round the first phase of the roads and tracks, noting the position of the kilometre markers, compulsory checkpoints and any places where time may be lost or gained. They then walk the steeplechase noting where the halfway or minute markers are on the course. They are finally driven round the rest of the roads and tracks. At a three-day event the rider would walk the cross-country course a minimum of three times, while at a one-day event the course would normally only be walked once unless the rider wanted to reappraise a fence. If possible the course should be walked at the same time of day that it is to jumped so that the rider is not taken by surprise by the position of the sun. If the rider has walked the course the day before but the weather has been bad overnight, the course should be walked again to assess how much the ground has altered; it may be necessary to consider alternative routes to or between fences.

At each fence the rider must bear in mind:

- how the horse will perceive the fence, for example jumping from light into dark;
- whether the approach is uphill or downhill;
- whether there is any rough or uneven ground to avoid;
- which way the ground falls away;
- whether there is a landmark to help the rider find the line;
- what influence a fence will have on the next.

Combination fences need to be looked at from every angle before deciding on the line that is most suitable for horse and rider. Having found a suitable line the rider should walk back from the fence to make sure that he or she can pick up the line of approach from some distance from the fence. During the competition the horse will be travelling quite quickly and so the rider must prepare early enough for each fence. The rider must consider the pace, speed and balance of the horse on the approach and consider the alterations that will need to be made after the horse has landed over the first element in order to be able to jump through the rest of the combination. It is vital to walk the alternative routes in case the intended route cannot be taken for any reason. The rider must bear in mind the consequences of crossing his or her tracks and take note whether the fences are numbered individually or are parts 'A' and 'B' of a combination; this will affect the way in which penalties are given.

The trainer's role is to help the rider choose the lines and options that will suit the horse best. Only someone who works closely and regularly with a rider can speculate on the rider's and the horse's preferences and abilities. The rider should learn how to use a watch at novice level in order to practise for three-day events; this will encourage good timing and judgement of pace. However, the rider should never ride against the clock to the detriment of the horse. During the competition either the trainer or the rider should try to watch earlier competitors jumping some of the more complex fences. If a route through a fence is causing a lot of problems it is worth considering a change of riding plan.

Show jumping

The course should be walked thoroughly, taking note of:

- related distances
- the measurements of combinations
- ground conditions
- gradient
- type of fence
- spooky fillers
- banners and other distractions
- where fences are placed in relation to the start and finish.

The ground conditions, gradient and type of fence will affect how the distances between combinations and related fences ride. The rider and trainer should be aware of the horse's stride length and know when this will need to be altered to jump the fences effectively. The rider and trainer should try to watch a few other rounds to see if there are any problem fences or if the faults are spread round the course.

To a large extent the trainer has to suggest a positive plan to the rider; if it goes wrong the horse and rider together will have to make an on the spot decision. If a related distance walks long only the trainer's knowledge of that horse and rider will determine whether the trainer advises them to move up a gear or hold the horse together for an extra stride. Whatever strategy has been decided, the trainer must try to encourage the rider to stick to it. If a mistake occurs the rider must put it behind him or her; there is no time to reflect on what has happened – there are still fences to be jumped! As the rider prepares for the competition he or she can mentally rehearse the round, visualising the perfect ride, seeing every stride, riding every corner and clearing each fence. With practice if the rider can hold this perfect image in mind, even if things go wrong during the actual ride, the rider will be able to keep cool and move onto the next fence.

Key points
As the rider and trainer are walking the show jumping course, the key points that the trainer would suggest that the rider looks at include the following.

The start
- Where is it located? Does this pose a problem for this horse and rider combination?
- Which rein should the first fence be approached from?
- What are the demands of the first fence? Usually it is designed to be jumped in an attacking manner.

The track
Between each fence the rider should look at the line to the next fence and ask:

- Does it require a change of pace?
- Will the horse have to make a flying change?
- Is it a tight turn or simply straight on?

Related distances
- Does the double or combination suit the individual horse and rider?
- Will they need to up the tempo and push on a little or will the fence require a more circumspect holding approach?

The finish
- Pulling up in balance is important.
- No matter how badly the horse has performed the rider must not overreact in the heat of the moment.

The jump-off course
When walking the course for a show jumping competition it is useful to note the jump-off track. If there is enough time this track can be walked and a careful appraisal made of the likely shortcuts. The rider should note the position of the timing equipment, shrubs and other decorations in the arena and decide if these will aid or hamper the planned route. The trainer and

rider can agree together what reasonable risks can be taken. Depending on the draw these plans can then be affirmed or amended as the competition proceeds. It should be remembered that a short track with an upbeat tempo, in rhythm and balance is most likely to be successful. A mad gallop and hauling on the reins may win one class, but will not do the horse any good in the long-term.

Warming up

The rider must be able to concentrate and stay focused during the warm up and competition (Figs 17.1 and 17.2). The atmosphere may be noisy, distracting or tense but the rider has to be able to narrow his or her field of concentration to just him or her and the horse.

Show jumping
A careful, correct warming up procedure can be vital to jumping a clear round, but the jumping in the warm up should not be overdone for fear of

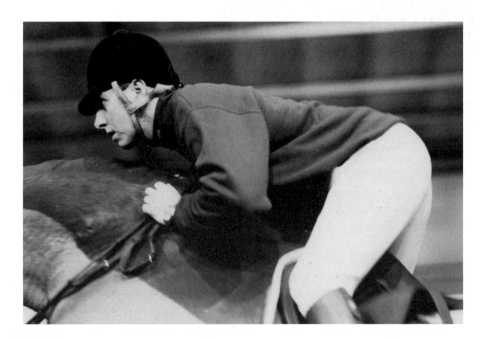

Fig. 17.1 Total concentration.

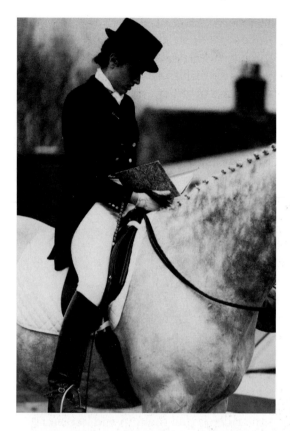

Fig. 17.2 A rider focused on the competition ahead.

'leaving the horse's jump in the collecting ring'. A total of six fences jumped off both reins is normally adequate. It is, however, important to establish the correct canter before starting to jump; the canter should balanced and rhythmic with plenty of impulsion. The rider should ensure that he or she can move up and down a gear in the canter and that the flying change is established (if the horse is of that level of experience).

Normally there is one upright and one spread practice fence. There may also be a permanent cross pole. Certain rules must be observed (see *The British Show Jumping Association Rules and Yearbook*):

- One pole only may be laid flat on the ground as a groundline up to 3 ft 3 in (1 m) in front of and parallel to the fence. There must never be a false groundline.
- At least one end of any other pole must be supported by a cup. Sloping poles are permitted on verticals and in front of spread fences provided that the top end is not placed higher than the horizontal pole.

- Unsupported ends of sloping poles must rest at or in from the top of the groundline.
- Alternate sloping top poles are not to be used.
- Spread fences must not have the front part higher than the back part.
- No pole can be held by hand for the horse to jump.
- Practice fences must be jumped with the red flag or support on the right and the white flag on the left.
- The height must not exceed the maximum height of obstacles allowed in the first round of the competition in progress.
- Horse Trials permit a 3 in height above the maximum height allowed in the ring.

Trotting over a cross pole first can help settle the rider's nerves and prepare the horse for the job in hand. It will also give the rider an idea of how the horse is feeling and the amount of warming up it will need. The rider can then move on to a small vertical to be jumped out of trot or canter before jumping a larger upright fence out of canter. Depending on the horse the fence may be kept small to give it confidence or put up to the maximum height to sharpen the horse up. The spread fence can then be introduced. With a young horse this would be built with a cross in front of a back pole before moving on to an ascending spread and then a true parallel, each with a clear groundline. The more experienced horse may go straight to an ascending spread.

The trainer should find out when the rider is due to jump and keep an eye on how things are going in the ring, letting the rider know how long it is until he or she goes. Ideally the horse and rider should enter the ring still warm from the last practice fence, having had time to check the girths and go over the course. There is nothing worse than being ready to go and then having to wait another ten minutes while all the adrenalin evaporates!

Cross-country (Fig. 17.3)

The horse will need about 30 minutes warm up before a cross-country round unless the horse is at an event where it has already completed dressage and show jumping. Depending on the interval between the show jumping and the cross-country the horse may only need 15 minutes' warm up. The horse should be walked for a few minutes unless it will not settle, in which case it can be worked on a large circle in rising trot until settled. It can then canter on both reins before having a walk. After this initial warm up the rider can work at increasing and decreasing the length of the canter stride to get the horse more engaged, active and attentive. The horse

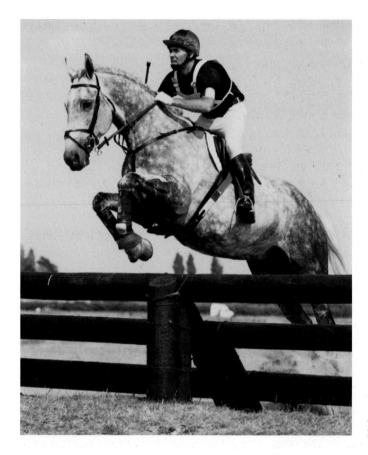

Fig. 17.3 Warming up for cross-country.

can then be warmed up over a fence; at many cross-country venues there will only be one warm up fence, often a log or sturdy upright fence. Initially this should be jumped from a steady, show jumping-type canter. Once the horse is going confidently the fence should be jumped from a slightly stronger pace to help the horse and rider find their cross-country rhythm. The idea is for the horse to take larger, more powerful steps without losing the rhythm and balance so that the horse can come to the fence on an even stride and jump it without having to alter its 'way of going', that is its tempo and outline.

The rider should not rush out of the start box and try to be galloping by the first fence. He or she should be particularly careful that the horse is paying attention at the first fence; once it is safely negotiated and the horse has found its rhythm the rider can increase the pace.

Pulling up

Once the rider has crossed the finish line he or she should slow down gradually, in a straight line and keeping a contact (Fig. 17.4). The horse will be tired and needs to be held together and looked after to prevent injury to tendons and ligaments.

Overcoming rider's nerves (Fig. 17.5)

To win, riders must be willing to take risks. If they make a mistake it is not the end of the world – in 6 months' time it will seem unimportant and in 12 months' time it will be forgotten. However, many people suffer from nerves at shows. They may be frightened of:

- failure
- making a fool of themselves

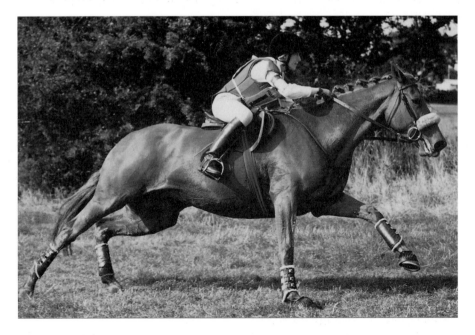

Fig. 17.4 When riding a fast finish the horse should be pulled up in a straight line and a contact kept.

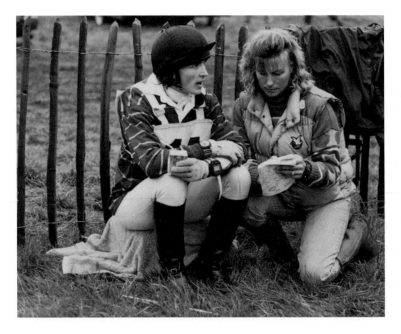

Fig. 17.5 Overcoming a rider's nerves by ensuring that the rider is fully prepared for the competition ahead.

- falling off
- letting the horse down
- letting the team down.

There is no doubt that part of the thrill of competition is dealing with and overcoming these fears. The trainer can help the rider by being positive and encouraging the rider to be positive and concentrate on what it takes to do well. When helping nervous competitors, take them back through the preparation for the competition to find out when the nerves and the negative thoughts start to undermine the riders' self-confidence.

- Do they demand too much at home before the show, resulting in poor performance prior to the competition?
- Do they panic because they are being watched by their family, the horse's owner or their trainer?
- Do they worry about what other people might say concerning their performance?

Riders must focus on the fact that the most important person to do well for is themselves. They must not run themselves down but focus on the desired results. Once their thoughts stray, fear seeps into the mind. The successful rider has to develop a way of coping with the inevitable pre-competition nerves. Stress management techniques can give competitors the power to gain some control over their reactions to pressure. Sports coaches refer to the athlete who is in control as 'being in the zone', i.e. the zone of optimal functioning (ZOF). An athlete who is in the zone feels good, sharp and in control of his or her pre-competition nerves. He or she is neither too complacent nor too hyped-up and are focused on the factors effecting success. The skills of concentration and focus can help a rider perform well even under intense pressure. Such people who have mastered these skills are very single-minded and usually successful. They only focus on those things that they can control; there is no point in worrying about the other competitors and how good they are.

Relaxation
Horses and riders perform best when relaxed yet the atmosphere at competitions is often tense. The rider can practise relaxation exercises at home, for example deep breathing exercises to reduce tension.

Centering
Centering is a breathing technique which can help the competitor to reduce tension before or during a competition. It gives riders control over their bodies and allows them to dictate the level of pre-event excitement. Normally a rider can master the technique by practising for about one minute a day for two weeks. Thereafter the skill can be maintained by one or two minutes' practice a week. Riders do not have to use the skill every time they compete, but they have the confidence booster of knowing it is there if they need it. Whenever they feel too nervous they can use the technique to regain control. The technique is as follows:

(1) Stand comfortably in front of a mirror, with your feet shoulder distance apart and your knees slightly flexed.
(2) Relax your neck, arm and shoulder muscles. Smile slightly to reduce the tension in your jaw.
(3) Focus on the movement of your abdominal muscles. Notice your stomach muscles tightening and relaxing.
(4) Take a slow, deep breath using the diaphragm. Notice you are extending your stomach.

(5)   Consciously maintain the relaxation in your chest and shoulders. There should be minimal chest movement and no hunching or raising of the shoulders.

(6)   Exhale slowly. Let yourself go. Feel yourself get heavier as all your muscles relax.

Increasing excitement

Sometimes a rider may feel that he or she is too relaxed and not sufficiently excited; there are two solutions. The first involves mental images of success and victory to raise arousal. The second uses rapid contraction and relaxation of small muscle groups. For example, you may see a tennis player quickly and repeatedly clenching the fists.

Winning

Ideally every competition will be a 'win' situation, not because the rider has been placed first, but because he or she has performed better than the last time. Failure is part of the learning process. Losing is acceptable providing that the rider learns from his or her mistakes. The trainer should encourage the rider to celebrate and be proud of personal milestones and achievements; that way everybody is always a winner.

What makes a successful competition coach?

The following are all essential qualities of a successful competition coach and all coaches should work on these qualities in order to enhance their effectiveness.

- enthusiasm
- empathy
- skill at the sport
- skill as a teacher
- skill as a motivator
- knowledge of the sport and its rules
- patience.

Appendix 1
Excessive Use of Whip, Spurs and Bit: Guidelines for BHS Horse Trials

Whip

The whip must be used:

- for a good reason
- at an appropriate time
- in the right place
- with correct severity.

Good reason

The whip must only be used either as an aid to encourage the horse forward or as a reprimand. Thus it must never be used to vent a rider's temper – any use for such a reason is automatically excessive (which is a breach of Horse Trials Rule 44).

Appropriate time

As an aid, the appropriate time is when the horse is reluctant to go forward under normal aids of seat and legs. As a reprimand, the only appropriate time is immediately a horse has been disobedient, e.g. napping or refusing (but not after elimination). Its use, for instance, after a refusal when a horse has turned away and is several yards from the fence is excessive. Its use after elimination is always excessive.

Right place

As an aid to go forward the whip may be used down the shoulder or behind the leg. As a reprimand it must only be used behind the leg. The use of a whip on a horse's head, neck, etc. is always excessive.

Correct severity

A horse may be hit hard as a reprimand only. However, it should never be hit more than three times for any incident; and if the horse is marked by the whip, e.g. the skin is broken or there is a weal, its use is excessive. (Note: the rider is expected to know if the horse has especially sensitive skin and must use the whip accordingly.)

Spurs

Spurs must not be used to reprimand a horse. Such use is always excessive, as is any use that results in a horse being marked by a spur.

Bit

The bit must never be used to reprimand a horse. Any such use is excessive.

Appendix 2
Guidelines for the Inspection of Cross-country Fences

Cross-country fences are used for three main purposes:

* competition
* pleasure rides
* training of both horse and rider.

Most fences used for competition purposes are inspected by a competent steward prior to the competition, but there are some unaffiliated shows where this safety mechanism is not in place. Pleasure rides may have jumps that are not mandatory but simply a challenging option. Depending on the body running the ride there may or may not be an official 'course inspection'. Training courses are not always part of a riding or training centre and so may not be checked as regularly as is desirable. In these days of diversification it is tempting for a landowner to spend a considerable amount of money on the initial construction of a course but then not realise the on-going expenses, both in terms of time and money, needed to keep the course up to good safety standards. On the subject of the construction of cross-country fences, it is undoubtedly a good investment to employ a professional, whatever the purpose of the course. This person may be a specialist fence builder or an estate worker, well-versed in the safe and sturdy construction of fencing.

It is recommended that novice riders are always accompanied by an instructor when schooling over fixed fences. All riders should always have another person there in case anything untoward should happen. It goes without saying that both horse and rider should be adequately protected against injury. The rider should have the best standard available of helmet and back protector, while the horse should wear boots or bandages, according to personal preference.

The following guidelines are intended to help trainers, riders and those responsible for checking courses for safety. Just as a horse is only declared passed by the veterinary surgeon on the day of an event, the same must be said of course inspections. The inspection can be divided into several sections:

- the going
- the fence construction
- distances
- the surrounding areas.

The going

If, during the initial construction, permanent take-off and landings are incorporated then the upkeep of the fences is reduced and the fences are more likely to be able to be used all year round. Sandy, gravelly and chalky well-drained soils also tend to need minimum maintenance as there is less 'poaching' in front of the fences. The worst type of soil is clay, which alternates between being very deep and rock hard. This means that the poached soil in front of the fences tends to dry into holes and ruts which can be harmful to the horse. Farmers are well aware of the speed at which this type of land drys up, emphasising the need to repair the going speedily if the best surface is to be maintained. There are two majors recommendations here:

(1) Restrict the use of the fences in wet weather.
(2) After heavy use the ground should be rolled or harrowed as soon as possible.

The construction

Regardless of the height of the fence to be built, the timber should be substantial. This encourages the horse to jump well and increases the longevity of the fence. Care must be taken that holes and gaps are not allowed to develop in the base of a fence, where a horse or pony could get a foot trapped. The face of a fence should rarely be truly vertical; either the profile should slope away slightly or there should be a secured take-off rail. There should not be any protrusions on any part of the fence where the horse could catch itself or the riders hurt themselves should they fall on it. It should be remembered that horses do not always stay straight and do not always jump exactly where the rider intends. The rails making up the fence should be secured either by rope or wire in such a way that they can be dismantled should a horse get stuck on the fence. Stone or brick walls should have the top protected with wood or be smoothed off so that, should the horse graze the top of it, it is unlikely to hurt itself.

Banks

Banks must be constructed in such a way that they are really solid on top and will not collapse. On the whole a steeper facing to the take-off is desirable unless the bank is a natural Irish or Cornish bank.

Ditches

The take-off area in front of a ditch is subject to great pressure as horses are often spooked by ditches and try to slow down or stop quickly. The pressure can be reduced by having a take-off rail secured to the ditch; this not only promotes confidence in the horse but also stops the take-off crumbling and falling into the ditch. If the ditch is on the landing side of the fence a vigilant watch must be kept for the bank giving way or holes developing.

Water

Unless the landowner is very lucky and has a water fence that has a naturally hard and smooth bottom, the water fence will need to be checked regularly, especially if the water is murky and hazards cannot be seen. Unless the bottom is very well constructed holes may develop and these should be dealt with immediately. From the rider's point of view it is wise to walk through water before jumping in, just to be on the safe side.

Corners

The wide, unjumpable part of a corner should have a tree or something similar placed in such a way that it discourages the horse from jumping the fence there. Any multi-choice fence should be made as safe as possible by blocking off hazardous routes.

Slanting or diagonal rails

Any fence using A-frames, cross poles, etc. should have a reasonably wide space between the two sides through which the horse can jump. These fences are notorious for catching out the unwary horse and can cause a nasty fall. Certain fences can be hazardous and should be either avoided or built with great care. When building table-type fences extreme care must be taken that a false groundline is not created and the face should not be vertical unless there is a clear groundline. Triple bars and similar fences should encourage the horse to bascule and gain some height, not to jump with a flat trajectory.

Table 1 Guide to distances in combination fences cross-country.

	Bounce	1 stride	2 strides
Upright to upright	12–15 ft (3.6–4.5 m)	24–27 ft (7.3–8.2 m)	35–38 ft (10.6–11.6 m)
Upright to parallel or parallel to upright	12–14 ft (3.6–4.2 m)	24–26 ft (7.3–7.9 m)	33–36 ft (10–11 m)
Parallel to parallel	(not recommended)	24–26 ft (7.3–7.9 m)	33–36 ft (10–11 m)
Step up and down	9 ft (2.7 m)	18 ft (5.5 m)	–
Rails to step up	8 ft (2.4 m)	21–24 ft (6.4–7.3 m)	–
Rails to step down	8 ft (2.4 m)	18–21 ft (5.5–6.4 m)	–

Distances

It is difficult to lay down hard and fast rules regarding distances as much depends on the purpose of the course. The guidelines in Table 1 are for horses from 14.2 hh to 16.2 hh (147 to 172 cm). The distances are total lengths, including take-off and landing, and could be found when competing at Novice (3 ft 6 in, 1.06 m) to Advanced (3 ft 11 in, 1.2 m).

Surrounding areas
If the fences are built in a fence line there must not be any barbed wire, protruding fence poles or tree roots which would cause an unnecessary hazard should the horse go off line. If a course is inspected in the winter, try to imagine what it would be like in summer. In woods and copses branches and roots are likely to be a hazard. If the fields contain stock, particularly cattle, check what arrangements are in place for their removal when schooling or competition takes place.

Conclusion

In conclusion there are two main factors to consider:

(1) Good professional guidance on the initial design and construction of the fences should be sought.

(2) Novice riders should always be accompanied by an experienced instructor, preferably one who is trained and qualified.

Appendix 3
Recommended Procedure in the Event of an Accident for Those Involved With Horses

(1) (a) The telephone number and STD code of your local doctor and veterinary surgeon should be easily available to you whenever teaching or hacking. An ambulance may be obtained by dialling 999, but you will be required to give your name, exact location and some description of the type of accident.

    (b) When out hacking with a class always take with you:
- money for the phone or a phone card or a mobile phone
- a first-aid pack.

(2) Keep calm and use your commonsense.

(3) If you are riding, halt the ride in an orderly manner. Dismount and hand over your horse. Dismount the rest of the ride if necessary and safe.

(4) (a) Go quietly to the injured person.
    (b) Secure the loose horse.
    (c) Organise safety procedures for other road users if necessary.

(5) If the injured person is conscious:
- Tell him or her to remain still.
- In order that you may give full information to the doctor, ask if there is pain in any particular area.
- Do not move an injured rider in severe pain nor if complaining of pain in the neck or back. Wait until skilled help arrives.
- Stem obvious, serious bleeding by applying firm pressure to the wound with a handkerchief or piece of clean material made into a pad.
- Cover the rider with a blanket or coat.

(6) If the injured person is unconscious:
- Remember the ABC of care and as a first priority check the airway

259

to ensure that the rider is able to breathe adequately. It may be necessary to adjust the position of the jaw correctly and carefully and to clear any obstruction without causing the rider to gag. If breathing is inadequate, despite clearing the airway and correctly adjusting it, then mouth-to-mouth breathing will have to be started at the rate of about one breath every five seconds. Learn this life-saving measure and revise it frequently.

- If skilled help is not immediately available the unconscious rider who is breathing adequately must be turned as one unit on to the side in order to avoid the danger of inhaling stomach contents. It will be necessary to control the head, neck and spine in order to make the turn safe and then to keep the rider in a stable position with the airway readjusted if necessary. Learn this technique and revise it frequently.

(7) Remain calm.

(8) In the event of an accident to the horse make sure it receives attention.

(9) It may be necessary to send for medical help or to arrange for the rider to be taken to hospital unless quite sure of his or her fitness to continue. In any event, if there is the slightest doubt in your mind always refer to a senior member of staff or call for medical assistance. In an emergency dial 999.

(10) As soon as possible, but within the limits imposed by the circumstances, reassure the rest of your ride by your own calmness and self-control and continue your ride or lesson.

(11) Remember to make your report in the Accident Book.

Index